PAEDIATRICS, PSYCHIATRY
AND PSYCHOANALYSIS

How do children and parents shape clinical practice? How can clinicians learn from the impact of their patients upon them? How do we recognise if health care practices are adversely affecting health care?

Children's health problems can place enormous strain on both children and their families. Whether symptoms are acute or chronic, assessment and treatment can be confusing and frightening even when the illness itself is not dangerous. Understanding the impact of illness on emotions, relationships and development is an essential part of providing good health care services. For health care professionals it is necessary to understand how their clinical practice affects their patients and how this reciprocal relationship shapes good or bad practice.

Introducing key psychoanalytic concepts Adrian Sutton illustrates through detailed clinical studies how psychoanalytic theory can be applied in a health care setting involving children and their families. *Paediatrics, Psychiatry and Psychoanalysis* specifically describes the impact of the patient on the professional, how conscious and unconscious elements need to be taken into account and to what extent these can influence practice enhancing diagnostic and therapeutic treatment.

Paediatrics, Psychiatry and Psychoanalysis is an exploration of the central importance of the patient-doctor relationship and how the psychodynamics of this relationship are crucial in providing information that can aid treatment. It will be of interest to child mental health professionals – psychoanalysts, psychotherapists, psychiatrists, psychologists, nurses, paediatric practitioners and those working in social welfare and educational settings.

Adrian Sutton is Honorary Senior Teaching Fellow at Manchester Medical School, University of Manchester, UK and Visiting Professor of Psychiatry, Gulu University Medical School, Uganda. His publications span psychoanalytic approaches in child psychiatry, medical education and ethics.

PAEDIATRICS, PSYCHIATRY AND PSYCHOANALYSIS

Through counter-transference to case management

Adrian Sutton

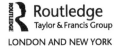

LONDON AND NEW YORK

First published 2013
by Routledge
27 Church Road, Hove, East Sussex BN3 2FA

Simultaneously published in the USA and Canada
by Routledge
711 Third Avenue, New York, NY 10017

Routledge is an imprint of the Taylor & Francis Group, an informa business

British Library Cataloguing in Publication Data
A catalogue record for this book is available from the British Library

Library of Congress Cataloging in Publication Data
Sutton, Adrian.
Paediatrics, psychiatry, and psychoanalysis : through counter-transference to case management / Adrian Sutton. -- 1st ed.
p. ; cm.
I. Title.
[DNLM: 1. Countertransference (Psychology) 2. Adolescent. 3. Child.
4. Professional-Family Relations. WM 62]
618.9289'14--dc23
2012033774

ISBN: 978-0-415-69265-6 (hbk)
ISBN: 978-0-415-69266-3 (pbk)
ISBN: 978-0-203-59112-3 (ebk)

Typeset in Garamond by
Fakenham Prepress Solutions, Fakenham, Norfolk NR21 8NN

TO DI,
OUR CHILDREN
AND THE PARENTS BEFORE US.

CONTENTS

ACKNOWLEDGEMENTS

We learn from, with and for our patients. The foundations of this book are their stories of health and illness: it is constructed from the material which they, their parents, families, carers and clinicians brought to and from the clinical process. In learning from our patients we become able to teach and be of better service to those who follow. Knowing this can, of itself, be of personal benefit to people in their illnesses. As I came to realise this more, I better understood the profound therapeutic implications of people having their altruistic longings recognised. I then felt able to discuss explicitly with them the use I could make of our work together to teach others. Rather than fearing that in seeking to benefit others they might experience a denial of their own needs, I realised that for many people this was a profound and often unexpected acknowledgement of their wish and ability to give unconditionally. For others it would not have been feasible to re-contact them to discuss this and seek explicit consent. Their clinical contact was at a very different stage of their lives and to re-appear as an uninvited guest, ignorant of their current situations, could not have been justified. I have used the *International Journal of Psychoanalysis* guidelines in terms of privacy and confidentiality. Real names have not been used and in some cases other disguise has been employed in telling their stories even where it has been possible to discuss fully with them the use of clinical material for teaching and publication.

The opportunities which arose in my training provided me with a multitude of inspiring teachers and supervisors. I was one of many medical students and psychiatrists influenced by Dr Heinz Wolff (1916–89): Dr Susanna Isaacs Elmhirst (1921–2010) had overall responsibility for my specialist child psychiatry training. They taught me that all medicine was built on respect for the individual and their relationships and that this was also the basis for psychoanalytic understanding. Dr Sebastian Kraemer has been a further key influence on my development, particularly in shaping my approach to the part the child psychiatrist can play in a paediatric department where resources may be limited and time of the essence. Their support and challenge to develop a disciplined spontaneity in clinical practice was reflected in my own experience as a psychoanalytic patient with Mrs Baljeet Mehra: her appreciation of the role of psychoanalytic understanding in child mental health in general rather than as a 'lesser enterprise' than its use in the analyst's consulting room has been crucial.

The clinical work described draws principally on work with medical and surgical staff at St Mary's Hospital for Women and Children, Manchester and Royal Manchester Children's Hospital. I wish to thank particularly Prof Sir Robert Boyd, Dr Stephen D'Souza, Dr Zulf Mughal and Mr Adrian Bianchi for the ways in which they made it possible to develop my role as a clinician and teacher seeking to integrate the contributions which our different specialisms can make to individual patients and practitioners. In preparation of the clinical material presented through this book, I am immensely grateful to nursing colleagues in the Surgical Special Care Baby Unit at St Mary's Hospital, Dr Michael Morton, Dr Liz Kaye, Kirsten Taylor, Lynette Hughes, Dr Jane Whitaker and Miss Cecilia Fenerty.

Inevitably in work with children, parents and families, one's own family lives with the ups and downs, the excitement and challenges of clinical practice and the turbulence of ideas challenged, changed and formed or re-formed. Writing a book turns out to be equally 'interesting'! It's been a bit like white water rafting at times; so thanks to Di, Chris, Clare and Emily for staying on board, bailing out, providing buoyancy-aids and helping me steer a course through it. And welcome to Betty who came on board during this last year: seeing the next generation and beyond confirms the importance of continuing to learn and through that to be able to pass on what has been learnt.

Finally, thank you to Angela Joyce and Lesley Caldwell of the Winnicott Trust for their encouragement and support in this project coming to fruition.

Adrian Sutton
August 2012

FOREWORD

As a clinician practising in the context of a general paediatric service, I found working closely with child psychiatrists immensely valuable. Adrian Sutton was one of their number and I have, as a result, read his book with great interest. The psychiatrists I had the pleasure of working with through diagnostic, therapeutic and teaching endeavours came from a range of psychiatric schools and each brought different skills and valuably variable perspectives to the bedside and the clinic. Adrian Sutton's approach emphasises psychoanalytic insights and psychodynamic skills. This volume thus distils the lessons which can be found at the interface between an analytic approach and the day-to-day challenges of paediatric practice; common and uncommon.

There are such lessons here for professionals from all those disciplines which contribute to the care of sick or troubled children and their families. Do we remember to consider that the patient's view of the professional is at least as important as the converse in many encounters? Do we recognise and use and manage appropriately our own personal feelings generated during interaction with the child or the family – the counter transference? Do we give sufficient attention to the developing psyche as well as to that of its soma? How well can we cope with uncertainty and, where appropriate, either leave a good enough situation alone or allow time to clarify the situation? There are many other useful thoughts, for example on supporting members of the team or on being an advocate in helping even young children express their fears or needs to, perhaps, a surgeon or other specialist.

The author is very candid in describing his interaction with individual children and thus exposes his thinking, sometimes about problems of almost unbearable complexity, to frank consideration by the reader. Few paediatricians may feel at home with every treatment decision described or every psychoanalytic formulation made. What is certainly true is that few paediatricians will fail to benefit by reading this book while reflecting on the strengths and weaknesses of their own clinical approach. I have found it salutary to do so. Those who read it will also be left with a clearer understanding of current and historical analytic thinking as applied to childhood. I certainly have been.

Robert Boyd, Professor Emeritus, University of Manchester

1

KEY CONCEPTS FROM PSYCHOANALYSIS

I'd rather feel stupid than be ignorant.[1]

Relationships evoke familiar and unfamiliar feelings. They cause people to act in characteristic or uncharacteristic ways. They shape and are shaped by what is spoken and unspoken, what is realised and what is unrealised. They may bring out the best or the worst in people.

Relationships occur in contexts which can shape how people think, feel and act. Context facilitates or inhibits the emergence of particular forms of relationships. In turn, different forms of relationship and context sanction or prohibit particular actions. The patterns which emerge create the possibility for a variety of thoughts or feelings to arise or fail to arise.

Patient and professional

Codes of practice provide a framework for practice which assist patients and professionals in knowing what it is reasonable to expect from the relationship. They describe principles which guide the range of behaviour which is acceptable from the professional but what cannot be codified is the range of thoughts and feelings which may accompany interactions. An essential part of professional training and continuing practice is learning to recognise these thoughts and feelings and to ensure they do not compromise the ability to fulfil the professional role.

Transference

Psychoanalysis emerged from the work of Sigmund Freud and Josef Breuer who explored the place of psychological trauma in producing symptoms of impaired physical functioning. Their paths separated because of differences of opinion about theory and practice. As Freud developed his approach, he found that particular patterns arose in the relationships with patients. His patients' experiences of him did not accurately reflect the person he thought he really was. When he reflected on their reports of their earlier, most important relationships he concluded that they were experiencing him in just the same way as they had experienced these key people at particular stages of their lives. He named this phenomenon *transference* to reflect the transposition of thoughts and feelings from earlier relationships to the current relationship with him:

> We mean a transference of feelings on to the person of the doctor, since we do not believe that the situation in the treatment could justify the development of such feelings. We suspect, on the contrary, that the whole readiness for these feelings is derived from elsewhere, that they were already prepared in the patient and, upon the opportunity offered by the analytic treatment, are transferred on to the person of the doctor.
>
> (Freud S. 1927: 194)

Crucially Freud's reflections led him to recognise and accept what was happening for what it was. He did not take it personally, regardless of whether it was complimentary or denigratory. It was a response to him in this particular professional role and emerged because of the particular form and structure of this relationship.

Initially Freud viewed transference as an obstruction to the 'real' work of the psychoanalytic process. His approach was more akin to an intellectual, archaeological process, i.e. the identification of the underlying events, experiences, impulses and their buried roots in infancy and childhood. However as psychoanalytic practice and theory evolved it became apparent that, rather than being an obstacle, this *resistance* was a mechanism through which therapeutic change could occur. The peculiar form of the relationship with the psychoanalyst, with its regularity, physical arrangement and disciplined focus on its aims and objectives, produced a particular constellation. The difficulties from the original relationship were recreated and re-enacted in the consulting room: Freud called this *transference neurosis*. However, this was not an arcane exercise in creating a false world for its own sake. What became apparent was that the symptoms which had led the patients to seek help were significantly contributed to by these same processes operating in their everyday relationships. This was leading to distress and dysfunction.

The realisation of the occurrence of transference, its acknowledgement with the patient and the identification of its effects in their everyday life became a fundamental component of the analyst's work with and for the patient. Juxtaposing historical, current and therapeutic relationships, with all their twists and turns, became a means of assisting patients to become less constrained by the adverse impact of the underlying confusions, fears and longings which they brought to relationships. Malan (1979) later captured this in his 'Two Triangles'.

By respecting the intensity and immediacy of the patient's experience of the analyst and simultaneously accepting the essential expendability of the analyst in their ongoing life, the analyst could provide an opportunity for problems to be *worked through in the transference*. What also became apparent was that the focus of the therapeutic process could lead to an intensity of experience in the patient which could not be contained in the consulting room. It spilled over into their everyday relationships, for example, causing an apparently inappropriate or understandable reaction to something or someone. This is the origin of the phrase *acting out* which originally meant the enactment of transference issues outside of the consulting room. It subsequently came into use in wider circles and has become corrupted simply to mean bad or unwanted behaviour.

Wider application of psychoanalytic ideas made it apparent that transference processes are manifest in wider personal and professional relationships outside the psychoanalytic consulting room. They occur in the general psychiatric setting with clinicians and other professionals.

Clinical example 1.1

Mrs J was seen as part of the crisis management after her son attempted suicide. At first she came across as defensive and agitated, giving an impression of hostility. However, as the consultation progressed, she began to appear more at ease and the assessment developed the sense of a co-operative venture about her son's welfare. As part of the routine assessment she gave a detailed description of her experiences of abuse at the hands of her parents and other adults. She also told me that she was worried that she was going to be criticised now for what was happening with her son.

Her son had remained on the ward over the weekend and I arranged to see her again three days later. When I returned, Mrs J was again hostile and 'prickly'. It seemed to me that I had again become a threat to her. I thought Mrs J had probably unconsciously experienced my absence during the weekend as a failure in care and protection and that this was resonating with her childhood experiences of abuse. Just as she had had to rely on her parents, trying to trust that they would behave in her best interests, she had tried again with me and I had absented myself when she was in need.

I would usually have reserved interpretation of an acute transference process such as this to the situation of a patient established in psychotherapy. However, the intensity of her reaction, and its potential to severely undermine her son's care, made me decide to respond by interpreting what I thought what was happening.

I told Mrs J that I thought something had changed dramatically in her feeling about me: on Friday she had found me supportive, but now she felt the opposite. I told her I thought she was again expecting to be treated badly by me, just as she had been by other people when she

---

was a child. I explained that I thought these things had become mixed up and that she was confusing me with the people who had abused her. Although there was no further specific discussion of this, her demeanour changed and we were able to re-engage around the needs of her son.

Transference processes can be conceptualised as one of the forms of illusion inherent in the human condition. The misattributions which constitute transference may not hamper efforts to live a reasonable life but, if they do, a variety of problems can arise for the individual himself and perhaps for others. Disillusionment can help people establish or re-establish a better foundation for their relationships. This may carry with it the sense of loss and sadness which is conveyed by the everyday use of the word as well as being freed from a burden of frustration, expectation and demand. It is useful to think of this as a dual process of 'de-illusionment', becoming liberated from the power of its enchantment, to separate this from these emotions.

Countertransference

Freud (Freud S. 1927: 517) emphasised the central importance of practitioners being aware of transference and taking it fully into account in their professional responses: 'the transference is a dangerous instrument in the hands of an unconscientious doctor'. It is a complex and demanding process.

There is an inevitable paradox in the analyst's task of using an understanding of transference. Patients evoke thoughts and feelings in the analyst which cannot be other than their own experiences however familiar, unfamiliar, unexpected or alien they may feel. The analyst has to be able to accept these as her own, allowing of what it may mean about herself. She must also be able to consider it *impersonally*, something which may have been evoked in any analyst simply by being that particular patient's analyst at that time in his life and at that stage of the treatment. This is the *countertransference*. It may be experienced in working with children and adolescents even though they are still in the immediacy of the formation and transformation of the relationships which will be identified in psychoanalytic work with adults.

The psychoanalyst has to be capable of occupying two positions, considering both what she brings to the situation and what her patient brings. The former requires the development and maintenance of a particular form of reflective practice (see e.g. Mann et al. 2007: 595–621) to recognise the patterns of relating and responding which are characteristic of her. These may arise because of her own earlier life, or perhaps particular current issues, preoccupations or interests. They may be general responses or issues which arise for the particular practitioner with particular types of patients. It may not always be possible to take and maintain both positions simultaneously. The consequence can be the counterpart of a patient 'acting out [in the transference]', 'acting out in the countertransference'.

The same discipline is needed in the application of psychoanalytic ideas across different settings.

Clinical example 1.2

Mrs T was attending the clinic with her toddler daughter, Lisa, because of problems in their relationship. After a few sessions, she began to tell me about her own severe problems in adolescence which resulted in inpatient psychiatric treatment. She described her battles with the staff and her parents. She told me that her parents had lied to staff at times. If she protested about this she was never believed: her protestations were seen as evidence of her disorder.

I had a special interest in Mrs T's adolescent difficulties and their later effect on parenting. As the Parent-Infant therapy became more robustly established, I asked Mrs T if she would mind if I looked at her psychiatric records. She agreed without hesitation but I immediately felt and thought that I had made a mistake. The request had come from my own interest. Even though I had given considerable thought to it, it was not directed by a properly reasoned decision that this would be of benefit to Lisa and her mother. On reflection I realised that to obtain and read the notes would raise again an issue of who would be believed – Mrs T or the ward staff? I was recreating a situation and dynamic from her past relationships with professionals.

I did not obtain the notes. When I next saw her, I told her that I had not requested the notes because I thought I had made a mistake in asking. I apologised and explained why I thought I had been wrong. Mrs T told me that although she had felt free in giving consent, she had found herself feeling extremely anxious coming for this session. She was worried that I might have seen the notes and changed my view of her. We discussed this further before re-establishing the focus on the relationship between her and Lisa.

In the first clinical example, the ability to articulate the transference process in an *authoritative but non-authoritarian* manner was critical in re-establishing the therapeutic relationship. Mrs T (whose story will be considered in more detail in Chapter 4) required something similar. My error did not fundamentally undermine the therapeutic process because I recognised and acknowledged it. It became a reference point with Mrs T, giving her an experience of me as someone upon whom she was relying for help who accepted his own limitations and 'realised the error of his ways' in stark contrast to her childhood experiences. Winnicott (1963a) specifically comments on how there will be inevitable failures and that these are sometimes the route through which patients may find the means to manage things better themselves. His comment is not a call to complacency but an acknowledgement of the challenges faced and the need to be realistic about one's own abilities.

A fundamental tenet of this book is that awareness of transference and countertransference and taking them into account in professional responses will act at least to minimise the disservices we might otherwise do and at best significantly enhance our usefulness.

'Who's in charge' or 'What's in charge'?

When transference was first recognised it was viewed as a resistance to therapy in the patient. But what are the implications of using the word *resistance*? It may sound as if there is a deliberate, wilful intention on the part of patients to prevent progress in therapy. It implies that the patient simply wants to thwart or oppose the analyst. If this is truly the case, then the analyst needs to re-consider whether there is common purpose in the endeavour (i.e. a therapeutic alliance) or reflect on whether she has misunderstood or been mistaken in her particular approach at that time.

However, 'resistance' in this context does not indicate that wilfulness, in the sense of a free choice, is operating. Action may clearly be emanating from the patient but we cannot assume that they are 'deliberately' choosing a particular course of action or that they are necessarily aware of what they are doing. Even if they are aware, they may not understand why, nor, if only for that particular moment, be able to resist doing it.

Rather than the question being 'Why are they doing this?' we have to ask 'What is making this happen?' We need to consider that some other part of the patient's make-up, of which they are not aware or, at least, over which they cannot take charge, is significantly contributing to what is happening. Freud formulated these concepts in two complementary models. The potential for either *unconscious* or *conscious* influences to be significant determinants of personal experience and action is described in the *Topographical Model*. The idea that despite our best efforts or intentions different aspects of ourselves can take charge of our actions is formulated in his *Structural Model* (id, ego and super-ego) (Freud S. 1933 [1932]).

The psychoanalytic treatment situation is one in which there is a meeting of two people with minds of their own. They have their 'internal worlds' and can influence each other's experience through their interpersonal worlds. The ways in which these processes manifest themselves can be subtle and even insidious. The impact of the patient on the professional depends on both the patient and the professional. The psychoanalytic practitioner must be able to gauge what is happening inside him or herself in order to decide what it tells them about themselves and what it tells them about the patient. To know what is clinically useful and usable information, calibration is required just as it is for any other clinical tool. Whether it is done explicitly or implicitly, the use of personal experience in professional practice needs to be done with great care and circumspection. The more usual mechanisms through which professional training and experience can make this possible are not sufficient for psychoanalytic practice. For this reason personal psychoanalysis, becoming a patient oneself, is a requirement for psychoanalytic training and for less intensive psychotherapy trainings derived from psychoanalysis.

Defence mechanisms and anxiety

It is not only psychoanalysts and psychotherapists who are prey to counter-transference experiences. The theme of this book is that the impact of the patient on the practitioner is a key factor to be understood and managed if health and illness care practitioners are to be of optimal use. Making use of the feelings evoked can provide valuable information in clarifying diagnoses and formulating comprehensive plans for the patient's care. It is also imperative to do so if we are to decrease the likelihood of errors, some of which may have grave consequences. Simply by offering oneself in a professional role one may be on the receiving end of very powerful experiences evoked by patients.

Clinical example 1.3

I was at the Family Court to give evidence in a case in which child abuse was alleged. No criminal charges were involved but it was alleged that the father of the child had abused the child. The father was applying to have contact with his child who lived with his mother. Mother and child did not want contact.

Each of the parties was represented by lawyers experienced in this field. They approached me as a group to ask for some additional help. They told me that there was some quality about the father that each of them experienced which they could not understand. There was something unnerving and profoundly disquieting about him even though they did not feel physically threatened by him. They asked me if I would be in Court while the father gave his evidence to see if I could help them make sense of this and ensure it did not affect the proceedings adversely. His evidence was being heard directly before mine.

As I listened to his examination and cross-examination I found myself feeling more and more uncomfortable and agitated. The content of what was being presented included issues relating to alleged child abuse of an extremely unpleasant kind. The father denied he had done anything wrong. He dismissed there being any basis for the allegations stating that other people must have their own reasons for presenting him in a bad light. He went so far as to say that proceedings displayed professional incompetence, including by the judge. He did this without any apparent sense that how he was behaving was not going to be helpful to his case.

Mindful of the request from the lawyers, I reflected on what was happening to me in observing proceedings. The content of what was being said was unpleasant. What the children involved may have experienced was disgusting. However, I was used to hearing about these types of things and the feelings I was experiencing were not the same as those they usually evoked in me. I was soon to take the witness box. This always gives rise to anxiety in me but the feelings I was having did not quite fit the usual pattern. As the cross-examination continued I let other possibilities come to mind. I found myself thinking 'If he [the father] felt like me about what he's saying and how he's behaving, he'd shut up.' I also thought that what I was experiencing fitted with what the lawyers had described.

In discussing this with the lawyers afterwards I explained that what I thought was happening was a process called projective identification.

Projective identification is proposed as an unconscious mechanism through which experiences which fundamentally threaten a person's psychological functioning and sense of existence are managed. The threatening inner experiences are split off from the rest of the person's experience, rejected and 'disowned'. They are ejected into the external world of relationships, i.e. projected, and experienced as residing in another person. The threat is then identified as emanating from that other person. As part of this process, experiences are evoked in the recipient. The impact of these may even provoke action, sometimes of an uncharacteristic kind.

Projective identification needs to be considered when it feels like something has impinged upon or intruded into one's sense of personal integrity in a profound way without readily being able to give an account of why this has happened. The expression 'I don't know what got into me' indicates the profound alien quality of something having breached one's integrity. My explanation of this to the lawyers made sense of their experience and assisted them in the situation.

Projective identification is postulated as a primitive process, present or emergent at the start of life. Holmes (2011b: 364) describes it thus:

> Psychiatrists use their feelings to empathise with patients. But sometimes love, hate, fear, rage, horror overwhelm, leading to bad decisions... Babies expel difficult feelings into a 'bad mother', who then 'detoxifies' what the baby cannot tolerate. But sometimes, especially with an unresponsive caregiver, projective identification represents the only means of affective communication... Awareness of projective identification counteracts splitting and boundary-breaking, helping psychiatrists see their countertransferential feelings as manifestations of the patient's inner world.

There is debate about the extent to which the term countertransference should be used to include phenomena best explained by projective identification. Although they both include (unconscious) projective processes, the original descriptions of countertransference involve processes which belong to later stages of development as well as the potential persistence of the most primitive processes. For the purposes of this book I will use countertransference in what some practitioners may consider too broad a manner to indicate the general issues arising from the impact of the patient upon the professional through unconscious processes. However, I accept that the distinction does become more important in the discourse about more intense forms of psychoanalytic treatments and finer theoretical detail.

Projective identification has a particular significance in that it formulates a process by which a sense of being able to manage can be maintained by making something that is 'me' into 'not-me'. This may even evoke or provoke a response in that other person which may appear to an observer to justify the attribution.

Clinical example 1.4

Dwayne's aggression at school was unusual. Teachers said he was attacking boys who were bigger than him, and then complaining that they were bullying him. The adults could not find any evidence that he was being bullied.

During the diagnostic consultation I disentangled the following. He was afraid of these big boys even before they had actually ('objectively') done anything to him. However, his fear of them meant that inside himself his experience was he had already been attacked because of the fear he felt inside. My understanding therefore was that from his point of view his apparently unprovoked attacks were in retaliation for the attack he experienced simply by being in the same place as them.[2]

A corollary of this mechanism is that it can only function through maintaining the illusion that, as far as the particular aspect or quality is concerned, 'you haven't got it in you'. In Dwayne's case this might mean that he cannot even contemplate that he was the original source of the wish to attack someone or, indeed, anyone. This made it easier to live up to an ideal image of himself. But the process took on a life of its own, leaving him with poor peer relationships and the recipient of blows from other boys.

As well as projection involving aspects that might be considered socially undesirable, it is postulated that aspects of the self which could enhance functioning and would therefore be seen generally as useful, or even virtuous, can also be projected (see e.g. Hinshelwood 1989). Thus resources which could be useful for functioning and development are not available. In addition, mechanisms such as these require psychological work, albeit unconsciously. Taken together, the primary and secondary effects of projective mechanisms represent a significant psychological 'workload'.

A key message here is that reliance on primitive defence mechanisms may effectively rob a person of useful aspects of themselves. If they persist as major factors in psychological functioning they may produce major distortions as described in *Clinical example 1.4*. They may also interfere with being able to tolerate essential health care.

Clinical example 1.5

Julian was born with serious malformations of his genital and anal areas. He had undergone numerous surgical procedures and attended regular appointments. Julian had always found consultations with his surgeons difficult but he became overwhelmed when he was transferred to a new surgeon, Mr Williams.

Julian had extensive behavioural and emotional difficulties and was receiving psychotherapy. In the course of his treatment sessions I had come to understand many of his other fears but it took me rather too long to realise that a serious problem could be arising simply from the surgeon's name. When I realised this possibility I told Julian that I thought that he was frightened by the fact that the surgeon's name included the sound 'Willy'. I asked him if this was the case and he confirmed that it was.

The fears around his genitals, and his own fury about what he had to go through, had been 'translated' into an attribution of murderous qualities to the surgeon who was in fact a man with a very gentle and thoughtful manner. Julian was subsequently able to recognise this and tolerate being treated by him. His therapy helped him move on from his conscious associations to the name, the attributions which went with them, through to the previously unknown (or, perhaps, 'un-owned') aspects of himself which, through projection, had changed Dr Williams into a monster.

Fight or flight

Projective identification is one of a group of phenomena called *defence mechanisms*, which come into operation when there is a sense of threat. The common term 'fight or flight' captures two ends of a range of active responses to external danger which also includes physiological concomitants, for example increased heart rate which can aid preparation for action. States of anxiety can arise in the absence of any threat from the outside world and without there being any identifiable physical illness which could produce the same physiological symptoms.

Freud proposed a model in which there was continual vigilance providing automatic monitoring of the internal state. This did not involve conscious awareness. He proposed that internal processes could cause a sense of threat to rise to a threshold beyond which there would be major disruption to functioning. At this threshold mechanisms come into play to prevent the conscious experience of anxiety and any immediate disruption. These psychodynamic defence mechanisms draw on other resources in the person's psychological make-up to maintain a sense of coping and integrity. They also 'divert' the person into other modes of functioning or relating which may or may not help them in the immediate overall situation.

In the case of Freud's patients who had 'hysterical symptoms' (now referred to as *dissociative [conversion] disorders* [World Health Organisation 2007]), they lost use of certain physical functions, for example limb movements, even though it was possible to demonstrate clinically that the anatomical and physiological component parts to make functioning possible were all present and correct. An event in the external world does not have to be an 'objective' danger nor does it need to appear overtly dangerous to the person concerned for it to constitute a threat and to mobilise defensive processes. Freud felt he could account for the symptoms through there having been a particular state in which wishes, demands and impulses had come into conflict. As already described these mechanisms need not necessarily make for what would appear to be a safer outcome in reality and they may even lead on to other problems, for example paralysis of a part of the body creates its own dangers. The 'fitness for purpose' of defence mechanisms in this sense is not judged by their apparent use in helping the person in everyday activities but rather by their value in putting the person in a position where there is an internal state which is more manageable for the person's psychological resources.

Freud saw the decisive factor in initiating defence mechanisms as being the *signal of anxiety* subsequently termed *signal anxiety* (see Yorke et al. 1989: 1–19). The term can be confusing when one considers that defence mechanisms function in order to stop the experience of anxiety. The differentiation which he made was that an unconscious trigger activated by an unconscious monitoring directed activities in an attempt to achieve a state of relative equilibrium, *precluding* any conscious experience of anxiety.

> **internal conflict** → **signal anxiety** → **defence mechanism activity** → **restored internal equilibrium**

The loss of motor function arose because the wish to act in some way was in conflict with the wish to not act in that way: the manifest activity contained elements which expressed the wish to do both with the outcome of inactivity. This provided a state of relative equanimity.

A simple 'binary' state of conflict is likely to be uncommon. The model needs to be elaborated to include the processes of mental life where there may be any number of compelling or conflicting forces or demands, pushing and pulling in different directions. Even though they may not be in direct opposition, they may still create states of underlying turbulence. Turbulence in the internal world may reach an intensity which causes disruption and triggers 'signal anxiety'. Recognising patterns as *emergent* places us in a better position to appreciate that they occur without personal consciousness, deliberate intent or even any intelligent reasoning. Subsequent events within and around the person concerned may make it more or less likely that the manifestations will persist and produce cascade effects whatever the expressed wishes or fears of any of the parties.

Development and psychodynamics

Different defence mechanisms and different times

Defence mechanisms take different forms for *developmental* or *dynamic* reasons.

Developmental factors

Projective mechanisms are given a different emphasis in different schools of psychoanalysis. However, they are regarded as mechanisms which operate from very early in life, perhaps even from the start. They are primitive/primary processes, i.e. they are not derived from other defence mechanisms. Neurological and psychological development bring about cognitive and emotional changes which, in conjunction with motor development, give different possibilities for the ways in which internal and external stimuli can be perceived, processed and responded to. These maturational processes give rise to the possibility of different defence mechanisms. A 'more mature' mechanism is one that shows evidence of increasing cognitive abilities. It allows for responses to be based in more sophisticated appreciation of the outside world. The net result is an ability to encompass more experiences without major disruption to emotional life or development whilst simultaneously adapting to the demands of the emotional and social environment.

Anna Freud (1936) began the temporal sequencing of the emergence of different mechanisms and the submergence of those which are primitive, less sophisticated or not so useful. Her model describes age ranges at which particular defence mechanisms may predominate and how they can also be expected to become less dominant and subsequently less evident. Holder (1995: 324–46) provides a summary of how this was developed to contribute alongside other components of the clinical assessment and within the therapeutic process. Edgcumbe (2000) provides a more extensive overview. Its clinical application will feature throughout this book.

Increasing cognitive and physical abilities are not sufficient in themselves for more sophisticated processes to occur. Aspects of emotional development may become 'stuck'. This process of *fixation* can cause difficulties through its direct effect of producing a mismatch between the external demands placed upon a child in the ordinarily expectable course of development and their ability to respond. Fixations may also cause difficulties because they can create an imbalance within the child between those parts which are progressing more freely and the part or parts that are stuck. Even in the absence of external stressful change, the increasing separation of different internal components may cause its own stress and lead to manifest problems.

What has been described so far is a model which anticipates progressive change within a particular time-frame. For those children who have recognisable global learning difficulties, the same chronology cannot be expected. Given also that physical development may progress at the same or even a faster rate, it cannot be assumed that the patterns and processes will be the same as for those children within the more usual range. Sinason (1992) describes some of the specific theoretical and clinical considerations for these children.

Fixations may be overcome, for example through specific therapy or environmental adaptations. However it cannot be assumed that return to a more ordinary developmental trajectory can be possible for all children. In some cases *developmental foreclosure* occurs (Laufer and Laufer 1984: 181). This is a situation in which the particular form of fixation is allied with an absence of the structures which could maintain a sufficient degree of resilience and malleability for change to occur. That area of development becomes a cul-de-sac. The task is then one of assisting with optimal development through recognition of the person's strengths and weaknesses in conjunction with promoting personal and environmental adaptation to minimise potentially adverse secondary effects (see Chapter 6).

Dynamic factors

Although the expectation is of a path which is recognisable as progressive when viewed across its breadth, the psychoanalytic model recognises that there can be movement in the other direction, i.e. *regression*. Regression is a part of the ordinary range of development and may at times be part of a process through which 'catching up' between imbalances in development may become possible. It can occur acutely or in more prolonged forms but with the possibility of regaining previous levels of functioning. It becomes clinically significant when it is persistent and/or becomes a problem for the child himself or for his carers. Differentiating between who has the problem with it in terms of the diagnostic significance can be complicated.

The particular form of the psychoanalytic treatment setting provides opportunities in which alterations in states of functioning can be observed, examined and their responsiveness to internal and interpersonal influences monitored. Meltzer (1967) described two aspects of the psychoanalyst's task being *modulation* and *modification*. Modification refers to the process of beneficial and lasting alterations in the internal world of the patient: ultimately this occurs through the engagement of the analyst and the patient in the exploration and interpretation of the patient's mental life. At times in the course of treatment mutual exploration and interpretation may not be possible. A variety of factors, psychological and physical, may influence this. (Physical aspects will be considered in Chapter 2.) The task of the psycho-analyst when the predominant factors are psychological is to respond in ways which can modulate the level of arousal to minimise or avoid any associated trauma for the patient with the aim of also helping them return to a range where the process of modification may be possible.

The analytic process requires the patient's mental activity to be above a minimum threshold. A sleeping or unconscious patient cannot engage. Above a certain level of arousal, changes in mental functioning may also cause alterations which make it impossible to engage in the therapeutic process. This can be represented diagrammatically (see Figure 1).

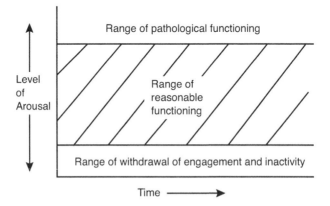

Figure 1

Clinical example 1.1 illustrates the application of this principle. Mrs J's anxieties led to her level of arousal rising to a point where the form of relationship she could have with me regressed. I responded to this with an interpretation which enabled her to regain her previous level of functioning. The following clinical example illustrates its use in the psychotherapy of a ten-year-old child.

Clinical example 1.6

Kerry had complex relational difficulties in conjunction with learning difficulties and serious visual impairment. In psychotherapy sessions she could vary from being impulsive, disinhibited and aggressive through to being thoughtfully engaged with me as someone whom she trusted or sometimes teased. One manifestation of this was in her sometimes being inquisitive and interested in my comments or enquiries but at other times being arrogantly dismissive of anything I might say or do. At more extreme times she could be bullying, threatening and even violent towards me.

In one session she kept insisting that I should not talk. Previously this had sometimes led to her hitting and hurting me but in this session there was a quality of mischievous playfulness about her.

As I observed what she was doing, I thought there were some important links which could be made about underlying fears, wishes and conflicts. However, I thought that if I made any comments directly related to these, it would be more likely to evoke at best unhelpful rejection by her and perhaps even shift her into a physical assault. Neither of these would assist the therapeutic process. However, I thought there could be actual therapeutic value in articulating something about the process of her doing what she was doing in my presence.

I felt that the response needed would be a complicated balancing act which did not place too great a demand on her. It would inevitably challenge her because it meant me asserting my autonomy by actually speaking and this would mean her being faced with her lack of omnipotence. The primitive mechanisms which operated in her meant that she could all-too-readily experience a lack of omnipotence as total impotence. Her usual defence against this was to engender a sense of impotence in others through projective identification. However, the fact that she was also inquisitive at times indicated an interest in finding out about things. This implicitly demonstrated a capacity to tolerate not being omniscient and omnipotent and a fragile ability to tolerate waiting to find out.

> I decided to simply say to her 'I don't think you're going to want to know what I'm thinking about.'
>
> Kerry was able to tolerate my comment. She laughed and engaged in thinking about what her activity had brought to my mind about her.

Kerry and I were operating at a borderline. On the one hand, she could be very easily tipped into a state of heightened arousal in which no therapeutically useful activity could occur and which could produce adverse effects. On the other hand, there was a possibility of her being able to tolerate the expression of my autonomy by simultaneously engaging with her inquisitiveness. I thought she had an *internal conflict*, between thinking she could be omnipotent/omniscient and enjoying the process of finding out more about these things. My response was gauged to try and engage with that playful mischievous part of her that was evident that day by making a response which did not demand a response of her.

In this situation I was conscious of the developmental gains that Kerry had made and the opportunities there were for further developmental progress. Simultaneously I was aware that her ability to maintain her functioning at its more advanced levels was tenuous. This lack of resilience meant that she could rapidly regress into more primitive modes of functioning, including into pure physicality.

The developmental profile

It was evident that when Kerry was functioning at her best, she was still not within the usual range for her chronological age. In addition, her ability to maintain her better levels of functioning was limited. Her comprehensive assessment involved obtaining a full account of all aspects of her social, emotional, behavioural and cognitive development and her social and educational situation.

Anna Freud (1965) described a comprehensive approach to assessment, developed further in the work of the Anna Freud Centre formalised in the *Diagnostic Profile* which is also referred to as the *Developmental Profile*. It uses information from clinical interviews with children and their carers, observational information and further information relating to cognitive development and physical health. This provides a 'snapshot' of the child in their developmental ability, inability, disability and potential vulnerability and a sense of the balance between different factors in their internal world. It also utilises the historical account of their development.

The psychoanalytic model conceptualises the mind as a system with different components which drive towards action and others towards inhibition of action. Some appear to be governed by 'laws' that one might think of as logical and others by processes that defy reality but do seem to have their own internal consistency. Survival depends upon a balance being achieved so that these internal processes operate in conjunction with the adaptations which are necessary to engage with the reality of the external world. The urge to take something into the mouth needs a counterbalance to say 'No'. Initially there is absolute dependence on the care of another person to be this counterbalancing 'No' to ensure safety but gradually it becomes possible to function more independently and take on more personal responsibility. Just as good coordination of muscles requires groups of muscles that, acting independently, would simply be in opposition to each other, so too does the psyche need a mechanism which coordinates and achieves functional and even graceful motion. Optimal development relies on the balance between impulse and its inhibition becoming modulated and well-reasoned. This involves a process of discrimination about what is essential and what is merely desirable and the ability to harness the forces involved to a state beyond reflex action and reaction.

The structural model of id, ego and super-ego was developed to take account of the different structures of the mind and their contributions towards personal experience, manifest behaviour and relationships. In simple terms, the id is conceived of as pushing towards action in a primitive, reflex way – the demand to be fed, the demand to have pleasurable rather than unpleasurable experiences. The super-ego acts to inhibit such actions. They can both be personally experienced as acting with irresistible force. The ego is that part of the mind which has to manage conflict between these (see defence mechanisms in the section 'Fight or flight' above) whilst simultaneously continuing the process of being in a world of external stimuli and relationships.

Reading about these different aspects can be complicated because the terms have come into general usage and different nuances have become attached to them. In addition different emphases in different psychoanalytic schools can be confusing. The id can be regarded as the thing which makes it possible to start living outside the womb because it makes us suck, get hold of the breast and be fed. However, an unmodified id would not make for a useful or fulfilling life. Maturational processes resulting in modification of this activity bring different mental experiences and 'accounts' of their experiences inside the baby. The decrease and cessation of 'biting-ness' on the breast may come from a sense of it not being necessary and from dawning awareness that it may be painful for the mother. It could also come from a route of fearing the process and the consequences of it, for example that there may be retaliation of some kind. This inhibition of action can be regarded as the first manifestation of a conscience, of taking responsibility for the effects of actions upon others and an indication of a super-ego having formed. However, the relative balance of concern, fear and the fact that the impulse to bite may simply decrease can produce very different pictures and lead to very different outcomes. An absolute embargo on action is like the imposition of an unreasoning tyrant. Hence, 'super-ego' cannot simply be seen as a 'good thing'. It is not directly comparable to 'having a conscience' indicating positive moral attitudes. Maturation should bring with it the likelihood of better reasoning abilities which will assist in taking more charge of the 'demands' of both the id and the super-ego. The energy and vitality of this can then be harnessed to support the child's development, gaining reasonable satisfaction from their lives and in their social environment. The ego is the 'virtual structure' which manages these processes. It negotiates between internal and external stimuli and demands, modifying them where possible and suppressing or deflecting them if they are disadvantageous, modulating them whilst simultaneously trying to harness their energy.

The term *ego strength* denotes the admixture of (a) a person's basic abilities, (b) his overarching ability to use these abilities in a way which maintains functioning and development, (c) his ability to recover previous level/range of attainment if there is trauma or temporary functional or relational loss and (d) his ability to adapt to changes in ability if he suffers permanent functional or relational loss. The latter two indicate that this is not simply a 'brute' strength. They indicate that *ego resilience* is an essential component, indicating how well a person contends with change that may be temporary or permanent, for example can a child cope with being ill or being away from home? Can an adult cope with the decline in their physical abilities as they get older? Anna Freud highlighted the importance of resilience in the face of loss as part of the human condition. Even with no 'objective' loss and given possible advantages coming with maturation, there has to be the giving up of desirable things.

Despite all the abstractions into the concept of mental life, the psychoanalytic model remains fundamentally a psychosomatic model. Mental functioning is necessarily affected by physical state. The ability to use one's abilities will be adversely affected by physiological and pharmacological influences, by tiredness or illness: the physical concomitants of anxiety may of themselves adversely affect psychological functioning.

In the ordinary course of events, neurological and psychological development means that different psychological mechanisms become available within children. In conjunction with an experience of care that is well-attuned and in the absence of significant emotional trauma, children develop more sophisticated ways of managing the demands of the inner world and of the outside world of relationships and learning. Winnicott captured this in the title of one of his books, *The Maturational Processes and the Facilitating Environment: Studies in the Theory of Emotional Development*. Therapy is needed where these inherent processes and the care that can be provided are insufficient or the demands placed upon children overwhelm their own resources. The aim of therapy is to assist the person to 'find it in themselves', i.e. his developmental potential, and recognise what is possible or not possible from himself or the outside world.

Imagination, phantasy and play

Imagination, the ability to form mental images and concepts, can be expressed through words, play and other 'creative' activities. The most readily identifiable items and themes of imaginative life and dreams are called the *manifest content*. Incorporated with this are other layers and facets, some of which may come to light through reflection and discussion. Beyond this can be multiple other layers or facets, the *latent content*. This latent content influences the person's mental life and behaviour whilst remaining unconscious but comes into consciousness if special conditions apply. The multi-layering and multi-faceting is called *condensation* (see Freud S. 1927; Laplanche and Pontalis 1988: 82–3). It is particularly evident in dreams, children's play and the games and pastimes of children and adults alike. The importance of play and creativity is captured by them being called 're[-]creational activities'. For example, conflict and competition may be an essential component. The wish or need to win may be seen as a manifestation of primitive issues relating to kicking or being kicked, being still or in motion, or even killing or being killed.

Imagining may lead to the emergence of coherent themes, i.e. fantasising. A story might be a single, one-off narrative. Alternatively, stories or themes in stories may be consistently repeated. These themes may be characteristic of a particular person and they may become an organising feature in their lives. When they are shared across groups and wider society, fairy tales, myths and legends can follow.

Seeking to understand unconscious organising themes (*unconscious phantasy*) is a key component of psychoanalytic treatment. In this area of mental life the rules which apply are either fundamentally primitive or only partially modified by experience and the usual cognitive maturational processes.

The psychoanalytic setting is one of those 'special conditions' where unconscious fantasies can become conscious. Through meticulous observation and attention, themes and patterns are recognised, articulated and interpreted. Bringing them into the light of day, the realm of more advanced areas of ego-functioning, their hold in the person's life can be realised, challenged and, hopefully, if they are undermining for that person, loosened or modified. They can occupy a different place, perhaps being integrated through re-working and *sublimation* (see below). The monster under the bed can be befriended and realised as fearful rather than fearsome: afraid as well as fierce; a complex creature full of contradictory wishes and fears; an external representation of the child himself. In considering the experience of bodily sensations and functions, later in the book, it will be seen how the confusions and complexity of somatic life and psychical experience are manifest in the paediatric setting.

Some psychoanalytic writings concern themselves substantially with the area of unconscious fantasy and its impact on daily life. Couched in terms of primitive (infantile) processes, formulations can seem bizarre or incomprehensible to the non-psychoanalytic reader, particularly when related to the mental life of adults. The combinations and associations, the themes, causes and consequences of events are far removed from mature, 'logical' thinking. They can occur in a particularly 'pure' form in the treatment and care of children with severe disorders.

Clinical example 1.7

Elizabeth (11 years) had been identified as having a complex developmental disorder which included bizarre behaviour and was being treated in a residential psychiatric unit. It had not been possible to establish a satisfactory diagnostic formulation. Her treatment in the unit was a combination of specialised therapeutic care, education based on the principles of fundamental (functional) learning and psychotherapy.

It had long been suspected that Elizabeth experienced hallucinations but she had never spoken of these. In session 15, she was having problems making something. Each setback was greeted with a shrill squeal. She banged her head on the windowsill and responded by biting the wood. I said to her that she seemed to feel someone was doing things deliberately to her. She replied: 'Yes. The Fucking Poo Boy'. This turned out to be an hallucinatory presence who denigrated and abused her. Soon other characters appeared –'Fucking Cow', 'Fucking Bitch' – and still more featured in her later enactments and play.

On meeting me one day, Elizabeth asked: 'Can I go up and get another jumper on?' 1 told her that I thought she would be warm enough with just one jumper. It was only later that I realised she could have meant a *different* jumper rather than an additional one! It transpired that the first jumper was her sister's and she feared I might think she was her sister.

In the subsequent therapy session, Elizabeth drew some fish and cut them out. They were put in a container in some water. When she held this outside the window, I was vividly reminded of her prematurity and how she had been in an incubator, separated by glass. I put something of this into words. Elizabeth then brought the container in, but 'accidentally' spilt one of the fish out. I felt almost physically hit by the phrase 'like a fish out of water', fully realising it meant fighting for life outside one's own natural environment. This was Elizabeth's experience physically in that early period of life and emotionally all her life. We talked about this and she then rushed out to the toilet to urinate and defecate in an attempt to expel her terror.[3]

In the more ordinary course of events the new mental mechanisms which arise provide tools that assist the non-disruptive expression of persisting primitive processes. *Symbolisation* allows their expression through representation in forms which can be incorporated into everyday life. Allied to this is *sublimation* which harnesses and channels the energy and vitality of the primitive processes 'under the direction of' more mature ego functions. This makes it possible to use this energy in support of productive or pleasurable activity or at least into non-productive activity which is neither disruptive to the individual nor to the community in general.

The outcomes of symbolisation and sublimation can be socially and personally acceptable (ego-syntonic) but may also contribute positively to the person's life and to others' lives. But when they break down, the consequences can be catastrophic. Segal wrote a classic paper in which she described the place of playing music in two violinists' lives:

> Patient A was a schizophrenic in a mental hospital. [When] asked by his doctor why he had stopped playing the violin since his illness [he] replied... 'Why? Do you expect me to masturbate in public?' ... [P]atient B dreamed one night that he and a young girl were playing a violin duet. He had associations [...] from which it emerged clearly that the violin represented his genitals and playing the violin represented a masturbatory phantasy of a relation with the girl ... For A, the violin had become so completely equated with his genital that to touch it became impossible. For B, playing the violin in his waking life was an important sublimation.
>
> (Segal 1981: 49–50).

Soccer, the 'Beautiful Game', can be a means through which impulses and fantasies can be experienced and find expression for players, spectators and associated other people. When healthy processes of symbolisation and sublimation are operating, this happens in a properly contained way. Responding to a question about an up-coming game, the football manager Bill Shankly quipped, 'some people think football is a matter of life and death. I can assure them it is much more important than that' (Knowles 2004: 724). His wry riposte captured the raw passion and illogicality that lies beneath and which needs to be contained in and by the stadium and its associated paraphernalia. When healthy processes have not remained in control, people have been injured and killed.

The emergence of symbolisation and sublimation can be seen in the psychotherapy of younger children in particular.

Clinical example 1.8

Terry was five years old and well-established in psychotherapy. He used drawing and modelling materials, toys and furniture in the room freely.

He would often play without talking much but he did engage with any comments I made. Themes relating to what can be inside or outside had been a regular feature. This was linked with his relationships and bodily functions.

One day he was playing with a toy, saying it was a plane dropping bombs. In context of other things he had been doing and which we had talked about, and in relation to his presenting symptoms, a specific idea formed in my mind. I thought he was both enacting a plane dropping a bomb and thinking about defecation.

I said to Terry 'I think you're thinking about poo.'

He replied 'How did you know?'

I explained to him why I had thought this was what was happening but that it was not because I could get inside his head and read his mind.

Some months later Terry's mother was nearing the end of her pregnancy; this was a major issue for Terry. In one session he was playing a game in which he was on an island and then on a boat. While he was doing this he was also drinking water. I thought that this linked with the themes of what could be inside, outside or on the surface of something or someone else. The boat and the island were on/in the water. He was on/in each of these. He could then drink and have the water inside him.

Having watched his play evolve for some time, I said to him that I thought he was thinking about the baby inside his mummy. He acknowledged that he was.

A few weeks later he repeated the water game in a slightly modified form. He then stopped abruptly, looked at me and said, 'I suppose that makes you think about the baby inside my mummy.'

Taken aback, I was lost for words, and I think I only managed an inarticulate grunt in reply.

I was rescued by him saying in a challenging but playful way, 'Well! Tee-hee! You're wrong. She's be born already.'

Summary

Psychoanalysis is a theoretical framework for understanding both the internal mental life of individuals and interpersonal processes as they occur in intimate relationships, groups and at a societal level.

There is a complex, dynamic relationship between different aspects of the internal mental life which consists of both conscious and unconscious elements. Generally a reasonable equilibrium is achieved based on personal resources operating in conjunction with the resources of those in intimate relationships, positions of responsibility towards the individual and the structures of the community. Disequilibrium manifests as symptoms complained about by the person himself or signs recognised by other people. The developmental advances of childhood and adolescence produce more sophisticated mechanisms which emerge in a chronologically identifiable sequence. Delays and imbalances in development may occur and be recognisable either directly or through symptoms and signs in emotions, behaviour and relationships.

The process of being in a professional role can bring unconscious processes into sharp focus. This is manifest through transference and countertransference phenomena. These need to be recognised and carefully managed. The particular issues of bodily concerns and dependence involved in health and illness care further accentuate these processes. Psychoanalytic psychotherapy makes very specific use of transference processes as a medium through which therapeutic change can occur.

2

PAEDIATRICS, PSYCHIATRY
AND PSYCHOANALYSIS

I'm a doctor whose job is to try and help by understanding about upsets.[1]

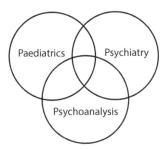

Figure 2

Medical Education has become an academic discipline seeking to prepare students and doctors for life-long learning. It has capitalised on research in 'Adult Learning Approaches' and teaching and learning methods derived from this (see e.g. Merriam, Caffarella and Baumgartner 2007). One such method is *Problem Based Learning (PBL)* (see e.g. David et al. 1999). It uses a structure which presents scenarios and defines steps to use in examining them. The aim is for students to describe what they think is happening, discover what additional information and learning they require, and plan responses to clinical situations. Its method involves ensuring a common definition of terms and use of language, brainstorming, hypothesising about possible explanations, prioritising the possibilities and deciding if additional information might be needed to come to a specific conclusion. A key component is that it seeks to mobilise previous learning and experience and to process it in applying it to particular problems in order to further enhance knowledge, skills and attitudes.

Although it is not taught specifically as being a clinical skill, its methods can be extremely useful if confusing or complex situations arise.

Clinical example 2.1

Sixteen-year-old Kyle and his mother had a complex and ambivalent relationship. They were very close but could rapidly become angry with each other. All efforts to improve the situation had been unsuccessful and this was interfering with his medical care for a chronic condition. A fresh opinion was sought.

The descriptions of the professionals already involved were rapidly repeated. Efforts to clarify issues with open questions were not successful in gathering a good history so I decided to ask for very specific details of what had happened that day starting with waking up. Kyle and his mother were able to agree that he had woken up and that he had got up and got dressed. However they adamantly and repeatedly disagreed about whether he had had breakfast or not. It felt like they could have carried on their disagreement all day.

In the spirit of PBL I decided to ask them to define their terms. Mother explained that Kyle had had a breakfast of tea and toast. Kyle agreed that he had had tea and toast but insisted that he had not had breakfast. He defined breakfast as a 'Full English' – egg, sausage, bacon etc.

It subsequently became clear that similar discrepancies occurred in many situations. This did not seem to be born out of any simple wish to be awkward but from some more profound issues about misunderstanding idiom.

Among other things this approach seeks to engender a true spirit of enquiry about one's patients and about oneself in relation to one's patients and other aspects of work and learning. It is a form of enquiry that is shared with the psychoanalytic approach.

Models of medical practice

Paediatrics, psychiatry and psychoanalysis have a common origin in medical practice. Medicine has provided fertile ground for the recognition of children's difficulties and for the needs of those caring for and educating them. It has assisted adults in understanding children, promoting their welfare and responding usefully to their problems. However, what has proven more controversial is the usefulness of different models of practice.

The Medical Model

The *Medical Model* (or *Biomedical Model*) was described by Engel (1977: 130) as:

The dominant model of disease today, with molecular biology its basic scientific discipline. It assumes disease to be fully accounted for by deviations from the norm of measurable biological (somatic) variables… The biomedical model not only requires that disease be dealt with as an entity independent of social behavior, it also demands that behavioural aberrations be explained on the basis of disordered somatic (biochemical or neuro-physiological) processes.

The debate still continues about whether it has been a constraint or interference rather than a facilitating influence on good clinical practice. It can be difficult to ascertain where the balance lies because it is recruited for the purposes of interdisciplinary dispute as opposed to rigorous examination of its value. Klerman (1977: 221) summarises this:

To psychologists and social workers in mental health settings, it is a term of contempt to use in the struggle over whether medical degrees are necessary for positions of greater authority or higher salary. To sociologists, learned in 'labeling theory', it refers to the narrow reductionism of conventional psychiatric thinking that refuses to see the social forces in the generation and perpetuation of social deviance. To civil libertarians, it is the basis for the unwillingness of the mental professionals to acknowledge the extent to which mental institutions are agents of social control.

He adds with added relevance to the present context:

To psychotherapists – medical and nonmedical – it is a synonym for biological treatments, especially 'shock' and psychosurgery, which threaten to destroy the minds and souls of their patients. To biological psychiatrists, proud of the advances in new drugs, it is a summary call to psychiatrists to return to scientific medicine and the mainstream of medical practice.

The Biopsychosocial Model

Engel (ibid.) views the Medical Model as severely limited because it ignores fundamental issues of the art and humanity of medicine. He summarised his objections under six headings:

1 An abnormality may be present, yet the patient not be ill.
2 The biomedical model ignores both the rigor required to achieve reliability in the interview process and the necessity to analyze the meaning of the patient's report in psychological, social, and cultural … terms…
3 Psychological and social factors are also crucial in determining whether

and when patients with the biochemical abnormality ... come to view themselves or be viewed by others as sick.

4 Rational treatment ... directed only at the biochemical abnormality does not necessarily restore the patient to health even in the face of documented correction or major alleviation of the abnormality...

5 The behavior of the physician and the relationship between patient and physician powerfully influence therapeutic outcome for better or for worse.

6 The successful application of rational therapies is limited by the physician's ability to influence and modify the patient's behavior in directions concordant with health needs... [this] requires psychological knowledge and skills, not merely charisma.

He proposed an alternative model, the *Biopsychosocial Model*, which would incorporate fully the science, art and humanity of medicine. Borrell-Carrió, Suchman and Epstein (2004: 576) summarised this model as:

a way of understanding how suffering, disease, and illness are affected by multiple levels of organization, from the societal to the molecular. At the practical level, it is a way of understanding the patient's subjective experience as an essential contributor to accurate diagnosis, health outcomes, and humane care... [whose] pillars include (1) self-awareness; (2) active cultivation of trust; (3) an emotional style characterized by empathic curiosity; (4) self-calibration as a way to reduce bias; (5) educating the emotions to assist with diagnosis and forming therapeutic relationships; (6) using informed intuition; and (7) communicating clinical evidence to foster dialogue, not just the mechanical application of protocol.

These authors do not present their arguments in terms of psychoanalytic theory and practice, but their tenets are consistent with psychoanalytic principles. There is a shared emphasis on reflective practice and the central importance of the patient–professional relationship as a diagnostic and therapeutic instrument.

Narrative Based Medicine (Greenhalgh 1999; Greenhalgh and Hurwitz 1998) is another approach which places these factors alongside biomedical evidence in the practice of medicine. *Values Based Medicine* (Fulford, Stanghellini and Broome 2004) also emphasises that practitioners need to be aware of their own perspective and how that influences the view they take of the data and information in the scientific literature, i.e. *Evidence Based Medicine* (Sackett et al. 1996).

What is good medical practice?

The foundation of clinical practice is the use of the clinical consultation. It provides the opportunity for the doctor to see the patient and the patient to see the doctor. Through this process necessary and sufficient raw data are gathered. These data are processed and formulated to indicate the likely possibilities in terms of health and illness (the differential diagnosis). It should allow the doctor to decide if further data are needed and what data are required to decide between the different possibilities. Simultaneously it provides a conscious patient with the opportunity to gain a sense of the doctor's trustworthiness, ability, and wish to gain an understanding of their predicament: explicitly it is the doctor making the assessment but implicitly she is also being assessed.

Through this process it becomes possible to proceed with a plan of care which both patient and doctor agree is a reasonable course of action. In emergency, the time-scale may be only the briefest of moments, but in most circumstances there are opportunities for repeated interactions, which may even extend over years. The presence or absence of change can be decisive in establishing the severity and danger of any symptoms or signs, in distinguishing between different diseases, in differentiating health from illness and in deciding on the usefulness of any intervention. Hence, time is an essential clinical tool for both diagnosis and therapy. It is also the means through which both doctor and patient can come to know the ways in which each understands bodily experiences, sensations and functions. Doctor and patient both contribute to the evolution of the clinical picture. Earlier clinical encounters shape the later ones.

The components of the clinical consultation are usually divided into two parts, obtaining a history and the physical examination of the patient. The history consists of information about the patient's immediate concerns, the background to these and the wider context of the patient's health, living situation and any potentially related issues. This provides the opportunity for the patient to say what the current problems are (his *symptoms*) and for the clinician to expand on this to explore anything that may clarify any additional elements relating to the symptoms or their impact. The examination provides the opportunity for the clinician to use their own physical senses and to explore indicators of health and disease, i.e. to elicit the presence and absence of *signs* of illness. This distinction between symptoms, what the patient complains of, and signs, what the clinician elicits, is extremely important.

Paediatrics and psychiatry certainly share the centrality of importance placed on this form of history. In discussions about psychodynamic psychotherapy, different schools may take different positions or emphases. Some may put more weight on the 'here and now' of the clinical encounter as a sufficient source of information; others on the wider emotional and relational context of patients or the historical events and processes of their lives. My position as a psychoanalytic child psychiatrist is that the framework of exploration of the patient's current concerns and predicament and how their relationships and development have unfolded are all essential. This should also include knowledge of the patient's physical health and development.

Psychoanalysis as a framework for practice shares with Narrative Based Medicine an emphasis on the way clinicians become part of the patient's life history: both value subjective experience and are circumspect about claims of 'objectivity'. The form which earlier clinical contacts have taken will shape how the understanding and expectations of health and illness have evolved. In turn, this will shape the form of ongoing and future interactions. A narrative develops in which doctor and patient are both characters.

As described in Chapter 1, what is distinctive about psychoanalysis is the position accorded to transference and countertransference processes as sources of essential information and routes through which comprehensive understanding and therapeutic aspirations can be better realised. Although psychoanalysis may at times appear to place a central importance on explicit interpretation of transference or other factors in unconscious mental life this may over-emphasise intellectual understanding at the cost of experiential and emotional aspects in the psychoanalytic process.

There is a further distinction between the practice of psychoanalysis as a specific form of treatment and the application of psychoanalytic theory in the practice of medicine. In work with children, the possible benefits of specially adapted care may also be underestimated. Winnicott (1953: 115) challenged his paediatrician and psychoanalyst colleagues to consider the place of psychoanalysis as a specific therapy as opposed to a method of informing other types of therapeutic care. In his 1953 Presidential address to the Section of Paediatrics of the Royal Society of Medicine, he presented the case of a boy where he had adapted his involvement to fit with practical constraints:

> Whenever he came to me subsequently he just played with the train, and I did no more psychotherapy. Indeed I must not, unless I had been able to let the treatment develop into a psycho-analytic treatment, with its reliable daily session arranged to last over a period of one, two, or three years... This child needed my personal help, but there are many cases in which the psychotherapeutic session can be omitted, and the whole therapy carried out by the home. The loss is simply that the child fails to gain insight, and this is by no means always a serious loss.

Psychoanalysis as defined by Winnicott was not available for any of the patients described in this book: some of the patients did receive *psychoanalytic psychotherapy*, a less intensive process but still characterised by the relative frequency of attendance and regularity in time and place. Most of the work presented is in fact *psychoanalytically informed therapeutic case management*. But experience and knowledge derived from psychoanalytic psychotherapy and psychoanalytic theory was no less important in the absence of psychoanalytic treatment in its purest form. A psychoanalytically informed approach can help us to understand why things have happened when there is no other explanation: it may help understand why something has been productive or counter-productive when there does not appear to be a 'rational' explanation. Perhaps even more importantly, it may help us tolerate not understanding at all.

The physical examination

The most obvious manifestation of the physical examination is the laying on of hands – the taking of the pulse, the request to open wide and say 'Ah', the stethoscope on the chest. However the first step is observation. Before laying hands on the patient, the doctor lays eyes on them: before any words are spoken, sounds may be heard; the entry of the patient may be accompanied by a smell.

Observation as a clinical skill is the readiness to take in perceptual experiences without necessarily being seen to do anything. These observational data may direct the clinician's activity and attention immediately: the obvious fracture of a bone, the smell of ketoacidosis, the sound of silence from the patient who has stopped breathing, will direct clinical activity urgently. Raw data need first to be assimilated without awareness of its significance. It requires what Keats (1821) called *negative capability*, 'when man is capable of being in uncertainties, mysteries, doubts without any irritable reaching after fact and reason'.

Examining the patient may include eliciting responses from them by asking the patient to do something or observing their responses, voluntary or involuntary, to requests or intervention. This establishes the base-line from which change can be recognised. Sequential observations over brief or extended periods of time indicate the presence or absence of change over time or in response to any interventions. For that reason there is actually no such thing as a 'negative finding' or 'no significant findings'; there are only 'findings'.

This process includes exploration and enquiry relating to mental functioning. This *mental state examination* is relevant across all areas of medicine and it is the specialist area of operation for psychiatrists. It begins by ascertaining if there is any impairment of consciousness, for example is the patient rousable? Does he know where he is and what day it is, that is, is he orientated in time and place? It includes assessment of cognitive functioning – is the patient able to remember things from the recent or distant past? If there is any impairment is it consistent or variable? Observations and enquiries are made about the patient's perceptual experiences, belief systems and mood. Is he experiencing hallucinations? Does he have delusions? Is his mood depressed, elated, anxious? Just as a surgeon may need to palpate and then exert some pressure in the right iliac fossa to decide if the patient has acute appendicitis, so too does the psychiatrist have to be ready to press and probe despite evidence of pain or upset. The examination is an iterative process. The clinician must simultaneously enquire and observe deciding whether repetition or elaboration is required in response to the way the examination is proceeding.

What has been described needs to be understood as the *present* mental state. What must also be appreciated is the extent to which this represents the state of the patient over time. Just as a patient whose blood pressure reading is high requires this to be monitored over time to find out what is happening and what it might mean, so too does a patient whose mental state appears abnormal.

Clinical example 2.2

Mary had been admitted to the paediatric ward the previous night after taking an overdose of tranquilisers. When I saw her for initial psychiatric assessment she sat silently and still in her bed. She did respond to my enquiries but only slowly and without elaboration. The circumstances before her overdose had given rise to concerns about her. She had talked about life not being worth living. However, the circumstances around the overdose had not made the clinicians already involved more urgently concerned for her safety.

When I saw her again in the afternoon she was sitting up in bed and talked to me at length about the difficulties she had been having. She cried during this but started talking about ways in which she might try and cope with her circumstances and get on with life.

Initially I did not know if Mary's presentation indicated a profound enduring state of depression or the pharmacological effects of the tranquilisers. By the afternoon it became apparent the latter was the case. If her state had continued to be the same as at that first contact, particular care would have been needed to ensure her safety and further assessment to establish how strongly she was in the grip of depressive processes.

Patterns of consistency or change may be crucial in deciding which specialist is likely to be of most value to the patient. Impairment of consciousness indicates that there is a significant organic process involved and that anatomical, pharmacological or physiological causes need to be investigated. Some common causes are drug or alcohol intoxication and diabetic crises. Less common are specific disorders in the brain or more widely in the body, for example temporal lobe epilepsy, systemic lupus, metabolic or infective disorders. Variability and lability of mental state indicate the need for exploration in the realm of physical disorder. This will be considered in the detailed case presentation of Jenny (*Clinical example 5.2*).

Liaison psychiatry

Recognition of the ways in which people's difficulties emerge and the ways in which this brings them into contact with medical services has given rise to a sub-specialist area of psychiatry: liaison psychiatry. It is:

> the sub-specialty which provides psychiatric treatment to patients attending general hospitals, whether they attend out-patient clinics, accident & emergency departments or are admitted to in-patient wards. Therefore it deals with the interface between physical and psychological health. There is now abundant evidence that medical and surgical patients have a high prevalence of psychiatric disorder which can be effectively treated with psychological or pharmacological methods.
>
> (Royal College of Psychiatrists 2011)

This definition has the advantage of brevity but it does not define what constitutes 'treatment'. Neither does it explicitly include the fact that a process of assessment needs to precede treatment, whether or not it arrives at a 'definitive diagnosis' on which a specific plan of treatment can be formulated and implemented. These points will be considered later in the chapter.

In child mental health practice, definitions of liaison psychiatry often extend to include additional activities which specialists from child mental health contribute, for example teaching, research and staff support. Different models of clinical services are also described:

> – *Independent-functions model*: the paediatrician refers a patient to the psychiatrist who makes an independent assessment of the problem and reports back to the paediatrician. Further action is decided unilaterally by the paediatrician.
> – *Indirect psychiatric consultation model*: paediatrician retains responsibility for the child and the psychiatrist offers advice and suggestions to the paediatrician.
> – *Collaborative-team model*: paediatric and psychiatric professionals work together to provide a comprehensive service for children and their families.
>
> (Engström 2002)

These models do not necessarily represent different *services*: they may describe different *functions* within an overall collaborative team. Hidden in this is also the opportunity to recognise a sub-specialism of 'liaison paediatrics' which assists child psychiatric practitioners in understanding patients' broader health and illness care issues.

This book is in the spirit of the collaborative team model. It describes a core function of child and adolescent psychiatric services as involvement with other health professionals when a child or adolescent has difficulties which involve bodily symptoms or functions. These problems may stem from, or be in conjunction with, identified physical pathology or may remain medically unexplained. Sometimes concerns such as pain, fatigue or loss of function may arise predominantly from the young person him or herself. At other times the reports of problems may preoccupy a parent (or other adult) to a greater degree than the child. The dynamics of these processes emphasise the additional importance of knowledge of the psychiatry and psychodynamics of adults for child health and welfare practitioners.

A brief digression into semantics and metaphor is required and will serve also to illustrate the complexity of this interdisciplinary work and lay the foundations for some of the later content of the book. The Royal College of Psychiatrists' (2011) definition describes liaison psychiatry as '[dealing] with the *interface* between physical and psychological health' [my italics]. But what is an 'interface'? For me it conjures up an image of a boundary with paediatrics on one side, psychiatry on the other. This does not fit with my view of the practice I espouse. The dictionary does offer 'a meeting point or common ground between two parties, disciplines, etc'. Strictly speaking a 'point' has no dimensions whilst 'ground' will have at least two dimensions and perhaps three. 'Common ground' is defined as 'something on which two parties agree or in which both are interested in negotiation, conversation, etc'. Liaison psychiatry does not necessarily bring about agreement but should be on the basis of 'common purpose' and acknowledgement of the professional abilities and resources of each of the practitioners. 'Negotiation' may focus as much on the issue of how action is authorised and by whom – my colleague Prof. Robert Boyd used to ask 'Who should be calling the shots?' Placing the clinicians in context of their usefulness to the patient rather than as administrative configurations of health and illness care services does require contending with greater complexity but it exemplifies a 'patient-centred approach'.

Rather than the relationship being one of 'interface' it is a relationship which needs to be much more in tune with the currents of mental life and their manifestations. As will be considered in the following section which considers the body–mind relationship, simple dichotomies are inadequate in complex systems. The ebb and flow of the different influences and expression of underlying processes are much more akin to the profile of the seashore – sea and sand with an intertidal area which needs to be respected for itself.

Diagnostic dilemmas

The debate between adherents to the Medical Model and the Biopsychosocial Model is reflected in the place of 'diagnosis' in child mental health.

> ### Clinical example 2.3
>
> At a case conference, the case presented was that of John, a ten-year-old boy who was brought to see the psychiatrist because he had been persistently pulling his hair out. After comprehensive assessment and clinical debate it was decided that the diagnosis was trichotillomania.

At its extreme in using the Medical Model, 'getting the diagnosis' becomes an end in itself; naming the constellation creates a state of apparent certainty: 'We know what we're dealing with: the patient is suffering from X'. However, as in the above example, a term can be as much a statement of what a patient does not have, for example some other state of being during which people pull their hair out. In fact trichotillomania is a *syndrome* not a *diagnosis*.

A syndrome describes a cluster of symptoms and signs which may have a number of causes: the clinical task involves seeking as much clarification as is possible in order to be properly informed and to properly inform the patient so the best form of action can be decided. The use of the term 'trichotillomania' does not suggest any reason, cause, range of prognosis or possible therapeutic interventions. However, one may find it being used as if it carries much more of the full meaning of 'diagnosis' in these respects. Its use may mask the 'not-knowing-ness' as much as the 'knowing-ness': it can create an image of knowledge and certainty rather than an authentic picture of familiarity, if not from individual professional experience, from the wider medical field. But this may all be another facet of a process which is 'a fiction of the investigator's desire to have simple answers to complex problems' (Blomberg 1996: xiii).

The converse, of assiduously avoiding the application of categories, can be equally unhelpful. It does not acknowledge the simple fact that there are clinical presentations in which common causality, presentation and prognosis have been established. In many of these there are reasonable grounds for recommending particular courses of action and not recommending others. Its use lies in the further recognition of what constitutes reasonable or unreasonable ways of proceeding. This issue of how to seek a language which has enough shared meaning and enough 'room for manoeuvre' in accepting uncertainty is a further essential strand in the fabric of this book.

Attempting to establish a diagnosis is more than simply trying to categorise disorder; it is 'understanding thoroughly what goes on in the mind and the body of the person who presents for care' (Lain-Entralgo 1982). The diagnosis needs to be considered in its relevance and use to the person to whom it is applied. The ICD–10 (World Health Organisation 2007) uses six axes of classification:

- Axis I: Clinical psychiatric syndrome
- Axis II: Specific developmental disorders
- Axis III: General intellectual level
- Axis IV: Associated medical conditions
- Axis V: Associated abnormal psychosocial conditions
- Axis VI: Global social functioning.

In child psychiatry, greater emphasis has been placed on the generation of a *diagnostic formulation* which is a 'working hypothesis'. It integrates the information available across these six domains to express the best understanding of the key factors and influences in the patient's presentation. Events subsequent to any interventions based on it may add weight to the probability that the formulation was correct. However, it may suggest the opposite. It may even allow us to believe *either*, since change in the course of treatment may indicate only that treatment has not prevented change, rather than necessarily having caused or contributed to it. The ability to remain open to new information and its possible interpretation is essential in order to incorporate this into an holistic understanding. 'Old' information must also be open to reinterpretation since change or no change can both constitute *new* information.

Linguistic dilemmas: mental life and bodily symptoms

The debate concerning terminology for problems involving bodily symptoms and mental life reflects the debate around the Medical Model and the Biopsychosocial Model. Lipowski (1984: 167) and Shoenberg (2007: 6) provide historical overviews.

Psychosomatic and *psychogenic* are two words in common usage to describe ailments when the 'mind' is thought to be a significant contributor. In 1984 Lipowski gave these definitions: '*Psychosomatic* is a term referring or related to the inseparability and interdependence of psychosocial and biologic (physiologic, somatic) aspects of humankind'. Psychosomatic medicine is

> a discipline concerned with a) the study of the correlations of psychological and social phenomena with physiological functions, normal or pathologic, and of the interplay of biologic and psychosocial factors in the development, course, and outcome of diseases; and b) advocacy of a holistic (or biopsychosocial) approach to patient care and application of methods derived from behavioral sciences to the prevention and treatment of human morbidity. (This aspect of the field is currently represented by liaison psychiatry and behavioral medicine.)

Shoenberg, 23 years later, succinctly defined psychosomatic illness as 'any physical illness in which psychological factors have played a significant role in its precipitation and maintenance and, in certain cases, in its causation as well'. In developing the ICD–10 originally published in 1992, the World Health Organisation had decided that *psychogenic* would not be used 'in view of its different meanings in different languages and psychiatric traditions'. It took a similar position in relation to *psychosomatic*. Winnicott (1989, cited in Shoenberg 2007: 1) accepted that sometimes words may fail us in our attempts to be absolutely precise but nevertheless they are the best we have in order to delineate a recognisable form: 'The word "psychosomatic" is needed because no simple word exists which is appropriate in description of certain clinical states.'

This reflects the complexity of 'trying to get one's mind round' the human experience of physical and mental life. It parallels philosophical debate about the nature of consciousness, for example 'Our normal awareness of space and consciousness is not geared to understanding deep theoretical questions about how the two things interrelate, but only to negotiating our world effectively. Looked at from this point of view, it would be remarkable if we *could* solve the mind-body problem' (McGinn 1999: 135–6).

The choice of terminology used sometimes implicitly accepts the practitioners' inability to find a physical explanation for symptoms whilst allowing of its impact on the patient, for example 'functional' to indicate that the presentation and consequence of whatever is happening is an altered ability to perform in the usual way. Other terms used may preserve the veneer of being learned and knowledgeable, using a term the lay person is unlikely to know, whilst implicitly being dismissive and denigratory, for example 'supratentorial'.[4] A major problem is that such terms can tip over into expressions which implicitly or explicitly carry moral connotations, for example 'putting it on', 'manipulative', 'malingering': *moral* judgements are a different species from *clinical* judgements. Clinical terms should carry information that indicates either an 'ordinary' range of experience and function or the acceptance of an altered expressed experience of the body or bodily functions and relationships in which suffering or loss of functioning occurs. The term *medically unexplained symptoms* (also called medically unexplained *physical* symptoms) – 'persistent bodily complaints for which adequate examination does not reveal sufficient explanatory structural or other specified pathology' (National Mental Health Development Unit 2011: 1) is useful because it denotes the clinician's position properly. It does not deny that the patient has a problem but it does also allow that the patient may have other symptoms which are explicable in medical terms.

Psychoanalytic contributions to diagnostic dilemmas

The description given in Chapter 1 is of a general psychoanalytic approach with specific reference to that developed by Anna Freud and her colleagues and successors. This approach is biopsychosocial in its appreciation of the variety of influences which contribute to children's mental health and the concerns of those responsible for them. Where differences may arise between psychiatry and psychoanalysis is in the emphasis placed on *form* as opposed to *content* in what patients do and say.

Clinical example 2.4

During a train journey with his parents 15-year-old Tony's behaviour and thoughts had become unusual. On arriving at the destination he had told his parents that terrorists were following him. His parents were very concerned and brought him to the hospital emergency department. During the clinical assessment he described other unusual beliefs which had developed during the course of the journey.

I felt his unusual thoughts were delusional but decided to explore whether Tony could think more about them and whether this process might give a better indication of how fixed they were. I asked Tony why he would be of such interest to terrorists. I told him I did not think he was giving me sufficient evidence to convince me.

After a while, he looked at me and said, 'So you're saying that you don't think they are after me. Well, if I believe you I'm going to feel like a right wally!'[5]

In the consultation, I had carefully attempted to delineate the nature of his fears, the possible routes through which they may have emerged, how firmly he held them, and how much they governed his behaviour. In the immediate situation I was not overly concerned with questions of *why* it was the IRA which had become the feared organisation or *why* this fear had arisen at this particular time, in this particular developmental phase of his life. My principal concern was not about the *content* of his thoughts in terms of any possible symbolic significance but their *form*. This was not to dismiss that there may be meaning pertinent to him which could be usefully understood in conducting any treatment. Given the immediate predicament, my approach was to attempt to assess if other aspects of his personal resources and functioning may be 'called upon' to create a safer experience for him. My aim was to try to create a space which was more contained emotionally in which to make reasonable plans for his immediate welfare. I drew on Meltzer's conceptualisation of *modulation* as opposed to *modification* described in Chapter 1.

I hoped to reduce Tony's arousal and anxiety through an approach which used challenge to see if this could help 'empower' his ego strengths to better contain the fears which had broken through. Briefly his strengths achieved ascendancy and there was the possibility of being in two minds, of contending with uncertainty rather than 'omnipotent' explanations of external persecution. The uncertainty was accompanied by insight into a sense of profound humiliation. Then his primitive mechanisms regained dominance.

Using Meltzer's formulation of modulation and modification there appeared to be a change in Tony's functioning which happened on leaving home. It became more intense and was sustained through the journey and the psychiatric consultation apart from this one brief interlude.

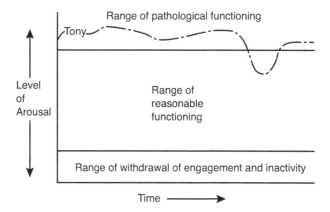

Figure 3

For a few moments Tony came into what I have broadly termed the 'range of reasonable functioning' but this was only sustained briefly. Psychodynamically it was not possible to pursue the idea of 'wally-ness' in its fuller significance to Tony. The balance was between feeling humiliated and feeling in danger from the IRA. The balance tipped back to the belief in an external threat.

This two-dimensional model can be useful but it needs further elaboration. It illustrates that there can be ranges within which different approaches to engagement may be necessary. Identifying these gives the clinician the opportunity to adapt her approach to the mode of mental functioning which is present in the patient and to see which aspects are predominant and persistent. This increases the likelihood of diagnostic accuracy. It also makes it more likely that anxiety or suffering that is driving the problem or secondarily amplifying difficulties can be at least partially or temporarily alleviated (see the discussion of *microtherapy* in Chapter 5).

Tony did fleetingly have insight. What became clear was that other 'forces' within him could override any other contribution that could be made. My position was to attempt to present a 'steady state' through being authentic in my responses – open to enquiry and testing whether or not he could be open to enquiry. I could believe or not believe what he said, maintaining my integrity of self without it being an attack on him. The affirmation of my own autonomy of thought was not an attack on him. Rather it was an attempt to engage with his. Simultaneously I was carrying out the mental state examination. The nature and manifestations of Tony's fears would be acceptably referred to as 'psychotic' across the field of both psychiatry and psychoanalysis (despite the frequent misunderstanding and even acrimony about this word between practitioners in the two fields). Psychotic states can produce profound countertransference pressures which can adversely affect functioning. Contemporaneously, I had to manage my own concerns about what I was going to be able to do given the resources available to Tony, his parents and to me.

The participant observational stance and perspective of a psychoanalytic approach provide a mental space in which developmental and pathological processes can be recognised and considered in relation to symptomatology. Regressions, fixations and imbalances between different aspects of development can be identified and contribute to the formulation of a more comprehensive approach to care. Psychoanalysis as a specific form of treatment may not be of use or may even be counter-therapeutic for a particular patient. But psychoanalytic understanding can help in directing clinical activity towards adaptations (in the patient, in those around them) generated from a deeper understanding of more realistic expectations and aspirations. This re-emphasises the need to appreciate that aspect of applied psychoanalysis which is a diagnostic process whose therapeutic value lies in understanding better the possibility and probability of dynamic change or developmental progress.

'Going over the top line' in terms of arousal produces a withdrawal from the influences of the outside world in as far as they might moderate some of the self-perpetuating, auto-catalytic processes which maintain or increase arousal and inability to function optimally. A different challenge presents itself when patients 'drop below the line' and enter states of withdrawal from engagement with the outside world and inactivity. These will be explored through Chapters 7–9. The countertransference pressures are very different. But when one enters this world one sees phenomena which again call forward the language of hallucinations, delusions, mood disorder etc.

The situations described all emphasise just how important it is that practitioners monitor and manage their own responses. A psychoanalytic practitioner will describe this function as *containment*. The practitioner's experience and functioning in doing so, or at least trying to, can provide additional and sometimes crucial information about the patient's state of being. Properly managed this can enhance the clinical process, taking it through countertransference to case management.

Demarcation disputes

The Biopsychosocial Model presents a case for integrating knowledge of the personal world of individuals and their relationships into clinical practice.

Medical education incorporates emotional, relational and behavioural factors within the domain 'psychosocial issues'. However, undergraduate and postgraduate curricula are not infinitely extendible so decisions have to be made about the depth and breadth of knowledge and skills required. Part of this is learning when the specialist knowledge, skills and clinical skills of another discipline, profession or clinical service are required.

Historically, clinical services and individual practice have developed out of necessity in the face of clinical demand, personal interest and ability: this gave rise to the establishment of new specialist disciplines, for example child psychiatry. As they evolve, clarification of roles, responsibilities and relationships is necessary. On taking up my consultant post in a hospital which had never previously had a child psychiatrist, a senior colleague told me, 'I think I'm going to be treading on your territory more than you are on mine.' He had developed an extensive, valued practice in both developmental disorder and the physical and emotional consequences of child mistreatment. His comment respected both his own expertise and the fact of there now being a recognised specialist training for child psychiatrists.

Contrast this with a scenario sometimes reported after lengthy consultations in which new, complex information emerges and throws light on the twists and turns which have occurred in a child's presentation. On reporting back, the response may be, 'Well, of course, I just can't have that amount of time to conduct a consultation.' Such a response implicitly denies that the clinical process and assessment owe anything to a difference in specialist expertise, although it does respect the fact that one of the most important tools available to clinical practitioners is time. The information may not be highly technical and scientific in its content and perhaps this is why finding it out can produce a defensive response. However, the knowledge base in knowing what is of greater or lesser significance, the clinical skill in conducting the process of finding it out and the attitudinal stance in integrating the information can be just as complex as those involved in the surgeon's or physician's activities. The shared task is to create a culture of therapeutic cooperation rather than rivalry in the service of patients, discerning where each of the defined areas of paediatrics, psychiatry and psychoanalysis may most usefully be applied for the patient's benefit, singly or collectively.

In considering 'pure' paediatrics, one might consider the child who presents with a rash, severe headache and a raised temperature where it is clear that the immediate need is for someone who can recognise and treat meningitis if it is present. For the child who is developing normally but then has repeated episodes of abnormal experiences including visual hallucinations, paediatric neurologists or neuropsychiatrists may be good alternatives in ascertaining whether this is temporal lobe epilepsy. The 'pure' psychoanalytic practitioner might work in a baby clinic and be available to help where difficulties are arising around sleeping or eating (see, for example, Daws 1989, 1999). A psychiatrist and a psychoanalytic practitioner might see their area of overlap or interface at its clearest where there is a youngster with a history of severe early deprivation. Ongoing relationship problems and episodes of extreme behavioural disturbance can give rise to the question 'Does this child have a "diagnosable" condition?' Is this a situation where physical investigations might provide 'objective' evidence, for example TLE? Might the situation be one in which pharmacological intervention can be beneficial, for example schizophrenia?

All parties may agree that the psychoanalytic practitioner does not need the involvement of a medical practitioner when they are treating a child with emotional difficulties who is in robust physical health and cared for within a resilient family. In the central area of tripartite overlap, there may be full agreement about the young person with severe anorexia nervosa needing, or at least, benefiting most when all three contribute. But these apparently simple boundaries may not stand up to closer scrutiny. The breadth of definitions given to child mental health services can be confusing. All children have minds and minders (carers, educators, supervisors of recreation, health visitors) so the possibilities of influencing their minds for better or for worse are manifold. Enabling good care, education and recreation is a service to children's mental health. But this must not be confounded with what is required when assessment or treatment is needed. Their service to the child is through their ability to perform within their professional role rather than through being seen as another arm of the specialist mental health services. Those other contributors to helping troubled children may themselves benefit in fulfilling their role through the provision of psychiatric liaison services. What brings the professionals together and holds them together is their shared responsibility towards children. There can be many areas of common usefulness for different disciplines, for example the acute assessment of children and adolescents who have attempted suicide where paediatric medical and nursing staff make possible the role of the mental health practitioners through their attention to the care of the child's body.

When considering referral, practitioners may ask how they should decide whether to refer to a psychiatrist, psychologist or psychotherapist. The answer is often more dependent on the ways in which services have emerged and on resources available rather than neat boundaries, defensible fully on solid inclusion and exclusion criteria. In the immediacy of clinical practice it has to be possible to make decisions about who is best placed to accept responsibility for action, for example the dangerously starved anorectic teenager, the acutely psychotic child. But in other situations this may need to be a process which in the past would have been described as 'trial and error' but which, one hopes, will best be described by its replacement term, 'trial and improvement'.

Where there is 'best practice' the process is led by the patient's clinical needs but it may become entangled with other institutional or societal issues and professional or interprofessional dynamics. Different parties may seek to write themselves or others into a role or out of having a role. Harrison (2009) emphasises how the models which are used on which to practice can be recruited for other purposes, for example financial. In his view, arguments for using a 'Biomedical Model' have influenced not only clinical processes but also the nature of professional responsibility, authority and clinical autonomy. In Chapter 11 I will argue that this may undermine good practice.

A further question for consideration in multidisciplinary practice is 'How well equipped are practitioners to recognise when they are presented with something beyond their expertise?' Mrs T (*Clinical example 1.2*), who is considered in detail in Chapter 3, presents a good example. In the course of the child psychiatric treatment it became apparent that Mrs T had had a classical puerperal psychosis after the birth of her daughter. Might these signs have been recognised if there had been a psychiatrist available (child psychiatry training in the UK requires substantial experience in the psychiatry of adulthood)? Her child's behaviour at two years old led a paediatrician to suggest and consider a 'trial of medication' of anticonvulsants. I was able to offer an alternative diagnostic formulation which was accepted and stood the test of time. This meant drug treatment was not instituted and its possible adverse effects (physical, psychological and sociological) were avoided. The recommendations for the treatment of attention deficit hyperactivity disorder in the UK (National Institute for Health & Clinical Excellence 2009a) state that the expertise for deciding when this should happen resides in some paediatricians and in child psychiatrists. Yet their trainings and ongoing collegiate work situations are very different. There may be major overlap in 'biomedical' terms but in 'biopsychosocial terms' there are major differences. The complex institutional and psychodynamic processes involved can provide very fertile ground on which enactments of unconscious processes can take root, grow and thrive. So it needs to remain an open question as to how much confidence should be placed in different doctors or other practitioners to know when alternative or additional factors may come into play in producing the clinical picture or in providing the best help to the children.

In practice it can be difficult to know how best to advise other practitioners how they should choose between referral to different disciplines within a child mental health team. This stems, at least in part, from the tradition in which I have trained – a biopsychosocial model strongly influenced by psychoanalysis both in the practice of medicine generally (Balint 1957) and in psychiatric practice. In addition to the influences indicated in Chapter 1, the influence of D. W. Winnicott has also been powerful. He was a paediatrician who trained as a psychoanalyst and developed his practice as one of the pioneers of child psychiatry in the UK alongside his psychoanalytic practice with children and adolescents. This exemplifies how child mental health as a specialism within the UK National Health Service, in contrast to Educational and Social Welfare Services, emerged as a function of individuals from different areas of medicine having the necessary opportunity, drive and interest. They also had the freedom to direct themselves into areas of practice, the need for which they recognised but which had not at that time been more widely recognised.

Do we need doctors to do the work described in this book?

The roles and responsibilities for which child psychiatrists are trained in the UK are described by the Royal College of Psychiatrists (2008). In fact the document defines more that other people have roles and responsibilities which psychiatrists need to know about rather than specifying the role of the psychiatrist. In reviewing these it has to be asked 'Do we need people who have undergone a *medical* training to fulfil these?' There is no neat, straight line which can be drawn between the knowledge and skills that are required to fulfil the General Medical Council requirements for preliminary registration as a doctor and the requirements for child psychiatry. The same is true for many areas of medical practice, including 'medical management'.

The challenge is whether other professionals trained at much less expense may be able to fulfil some or all of these roles and responsibilities. Some child psychiatrists have suggested a much narrower remit for consultant child psychiatrists (e.g. Goodman 1997). It could be argued that such a delineation is a 'retreat' into a Medical Model in contrast to maintaining an holistic Biopsychosocial Model. My own pragmatic position is that in everyday clinical practice the demand for the services of child psychiatrists as well as other child mental health specialists has continued to be greater than the resources available to respond. There also continues to be unrecognised unmet need. There does seem to be a significant belief from outside that medical practitioners have value in child psychiatry.

Simultaneously there can be persisting significant ambivalence about the speciality and towards psychiatrists. I was contacted by a lawyer for advice. She wondered if I could suggest the name of a suitable psychologist who could assess a child. I asked for details and she described a child whom I thought could very appropriately be referred to a child psychiatrist. I checked that the lawyer was clear that I was a psychiatrist. I then asked why she wanted a psychologist rather than a psychiatrist. She told me it was not good for children to be referred to psychiatrists because of the stigma. I asked why she had contacted me. She explained that I had been recommended because of my positive contribution in seeing a child for another case. She good-humouredly accepted my suggestion that she needed to examine her prejudices.

Some medical and surgical colleagues raise concern about too much 'touchy-feely stuff' at the expense of anatomy, physiology, pharmacology etc. in clinical practice and medical education. Their concerns need to be taken seriously if we are properly to balance the different elements of the bio-, psycho- and social of a biopsychosocial approach. Child mental health teams need readily available access to a base-line knowledge of organic conditions and this can be well-supplied by psychiatrists. We also need to ensure that the literal touch and feel of patients is in the experience of members of child mental services even if the practitioners are operating only in the area of metaphorical touch and feel. We need people who have handled bodies, healthy bodies and sick bodies which produce unpleasant sights, sounds, smells. We need people who have had to do unpleasant things to patients. We need clinicians who have been with people as they die. Working alongside other colleagues with different experiences, I believe can help build a culture for child mental health services which is fundamentally based in the unavoidably psychosomatic nature of humanity.

Summary and conclusions

The underlying theoretical framework which clinicians use can have profound implications for the clinical process. It contributes to the shaping of the clinical contact with children, their parents, colleagues and the wider professional, organisational and societal framework. It can make the difference between raw data being noticed and noted or unnoticed and un-noted. The emergent forms of understanding of the clinical picture cannot be separated from the clinician's viewing point and their ways of relating to data and relationships.

The tools we have at our disposal to communicate about our experiences personally and professionally can be simultaneously sophisticated and inadequate for our task if we think that task involves absolute certainties in understanding health and illness. The models we use professionally are tools which can help orientate us to our place in other people's lives alongside other professionals. Their usefulness is constrained by the extent to which we are able to know that we are using them and why we are using them.

Similarly, the distinctions between different professionals in their roles can be difficult to ascertain. This may sometimes relate to the fact of there being an inevitable lack of clarity derived from the nature of clinical presentations and the available resources. It may also be difficult because of the different qualities that individuals bring to clinical work from their professional origins, experiences and, not least, because of their personal qualities. This builds a complex picture of clinical practice with people in vulnerable situations full of uncertainties and the interaction of conscious and unconscious processes. The possibilities for unproductive and even counter-productive activity are manifold. Fulfilling their roles and responsibilities relies on institutions and organisation incorporating mechanisms to protect the central task of health and illness care.

3

FINDING ONE'S PLACE

If doctors are meant to be taught leadership skills who is being taught followership skills?[1]

Before giving some descriptions of establishing clinical relationships in practice, some philosophical and psychoanalytic contributions to understanding trust and trustworthiness need to be considered.

Finding one's place in the clinical world

Human relationships are not simply about leading and following. Sometimes they are about being in the same place as each other without the relationship being defined by anything except time and space. Sometimes they are about being together with shared concerns and common purpose. Contending with different relationships involves the development of 'knowing one's place' skills. In clinical practice, this means our place with patients, those in key relationships with them and our colleagues. The question posed above was not derived from a belief that doctors should be leaders. It was a challenge to colleagues to realise their place in clinical teams.

Finding out about our place in people's lives and their place in ours involves empathy: 'The power of mentally identifying oneself with (and so fully comprehending) a person or object of contemplation' (SOED). In the medical context, Zinn (1993: 306) describes it as

> a process for understanding an individual's subjective experiences by vicariously sharing that experience while maintaining an observant stance. It is a useful tool in the medical encounter as it provides the physician with a fuller, more personalized view of the patient, and it provides the patient with a sense of connectedness to the physician that may allow him/her to more freely express his/her emotional distress.

It is highly significant that Zinn defines to it as a 'process'. Making an 'empathic statement' is not an end-point after which one can tick a box to state 'I showed empathy'.

'Fully understanding' is an excellent *aspiration* but probably an unrealistic *expectation*.[2] In fact, more realistic is an ability to convey a depth of *appreciation* of the other, a sympathetic awareness and tolerance. 'Appreciation' may be present without true understanding and even in the presence of misattribution. Embedded in this empathic process are unconscious processes through which both parties are able to learn to accept and live with imprecision. Despite the best will in the world, there will be areas in which there is no understanding, incomplete understanding or even misunderstanding. From a psychoanalytic viewpoint, 'identification with' is more complex than the definition conveys. The psychodynamic mechanisms involved can achieve a sense of 'something shared' but it can also contain '*somethings* merged': this process may have contradictory effects – avoiding any sense of total alone-ness but denying individual identity. This will be considered later in the book (see Chapter 10).

The empathic clinician also needs to be a person whose actions are appropriate and in whom individuals and society can have confidence. O'Neill (2002a) believes that there has been a societal 'crisis of trust' including in health care. Different qualities may be accorded different values by each party in relationships. Trusting another person involves 'accept[ing] vulnerability to another's possible but not expected ill will (or lack of good will) toward one' (Baier 1986: 235). From the psychiatric and psychodynamic point of view we can expand the idea of 'ill will' to include 'illnesses of will, thoughts, and emotions'.[3] Such illnesses can set the scene as one of dis-ease and misattribution and lead to actions in the sufferer or those around them which cause further dis-ease and misunderstanding.

Trust and trustworthiness rely on a sense of not simply being tolerated but of being appreciated for the qualities one has. This is an acceptance of abilities, inabilities and vulnerabilities and being treated with *kindness* in the sense that it is derived from *kinship*, of having certain basic human needs and wishes in common (Philips and Taylor 2009). Trusting means expecting that others will respond to these, and take them into account in what they do even if the outcome cannot be what was desired. Health in relationships means accommodating and being accommodated.

Tony (*Clinical example 2.4*) believed IRA terrorists were seeking to harm him. He was in a hypervigilant state and behaved unusually. This produced concerned responses in those around him: these responses were frustrating for him. Briefly he was able to consider that he might be mistaken in his beliefs. With that came a sense of utter humiliation and a crisis of trust in the extent to which he should trust his own judgement rather than that of another person. Both scenarios were threatening but ultimately something threw him back to trust his own judgement of being in danger from the outside world. Tony could not continue to 'accommodate' an alternative view and to be in two minds. In responding to him, I had to appreciate his position and simultaneously accept that he might not think me trustworthy because I did not agree with him.

Most clinical practice does not take place in situations where there is such a profound disruption of trust nor the presence of beliefs of the nature of Tony's. However, in working with children and their parents, two factors need to be taken into account. Developmental factors mean that beliefs, actions and emotional responses that would be considered unusual if they occurred in an adult are normal in a child or adolescent. States of anxiety and hypervigilance can lead to regression to earlier modes of mental functioning (see Chapter 2) in adults as well as in children; this is especially pertinent in considering parental responses where there is concern and responsibility for their child.

Becoming established in the clinical setting

For any medical student, stepping into the clinical setting in their new role is a landmark event. It provokes a multitude of emotions including anxiety. The student has to manage these to be sufficiently at ease to learn about this new role and to learn in this new role. Along with being aware of what they have learnt, students will become acutely aware of how much they do not know. They face challenges about attitudes and values as well as knowledge and skills. They have to feel confident that it is legitimate to be part of the lives of patients upon whom they rely for their learning. What might otherwise appear a selfish pursuit of personal ambition is essential for all of us if we are to have doctors to look after us.

Becoming established in a paediatric setting brings additional challenges. Despite having been children themselves, it may feel like an alien environment. It brings with it the complexity of managing relationships with less assistance from language or presumptions of shared understanding; it also means always being involved with their patient and a third party. In response to this, I introduced seminars for students to consider communication from a developmental perspective.[4]

Students were given a brief introduction to the task which was to understand more about children's experiences of hospital and their modes of communication by spending some unstructured time with a child in the clinical setting. They were instructed to arrange a suitable situation for the meeting and to have some drawing and play materials available. If they did not already know the child, they were asked to have an appropriate adult introduce them. They were told to explain that they were learning to be doctors and would like to spend some time with them. No notes were to be taken while they were with the child, but they were asked to write down as much as they could remember afterwards and to bring their notes to the seminar. The aim of the instructions was to provide a general structure to facilitate while minimising constraints. Some students found the lack of specificity difficult to consider but were usually able to accept my explanation that it needed to be left open in this way to explore the subject properly.

Tutorial example 1

At an earlier tutorial on child protection, the student who presented the following material had already shown herself to be astute and thoughtful in discussion of a baby and its mother. She told us the mother 'was the sort of woman who, if you were taking a photo of her holding her baby...she'd be looking and smiling at the camera not at her baby'.

For the assignment, she had seen a five-year-old boy. She already knew him as she had been present the previous evening when he had been admitted with a severe asthma attack. He was now almost completely recovered. He was an intelligent precocious child whom people initially found charming but who had by this time irritated everyone with his imperious attitude. The student knew she had to prepare the assignment and despite some misgivings, she decided to approach him.

She introduced herself politely as a medical student, but he totally ignored her. She thought she had nothing to lose so spontaneously tried a different approach. 'I'm not really a medical student, I'm really a Red Indian squaw and my pigtails have been cut off.'

The boy stopped in his tracks, captivated. He immediately told her he would draw the person who had done it. During their conversation he developed the story, producing further drawings to say it was a monster who cut things off people. He went into great detail. The student and the child both took great pleasure as he spontaneously developed his story with this unintrusive, playful and facilitating young woman.

The seminar discussion considered issues relevant to five year olds generally. I proposed an explanation in psychoanalytic terms for the boy's response to the comment about pigtails being cut off, and his obvious fascination with the perpetrator. I suggested it stemmed from fears about bodily integrity. We discussed possible links with his asthmatic experiences. At the end of this I referred to the way the student had been able to engage the child and suggested that without realising it she had registered something important for the boy. I went on to describe how the feelings and reactions brought out in us by our patients can be examined to see if they may give us further information which might prove useful in assessment and treatment.

Tutorial example 2

Two students from different groups described a situation where the children they selected, a four-year-old girl and a three-year-old boy, had been wary about becoming involved with them although their reaction did not make the students feel they should withdraw. In both cases the children slowly responded to the sensitive interest shown and seemed to enjoy their contact with the students. In describing the ending of their time with the children both students independently and spontaneously said they had felt bad about it. They felt their process of engagement with the children had been in the form of offering a relationship but that in the end they were simply withdrawing, 'shutting the door'.

Tutorial example 3

An adolescent with muscular dystrophy, an intelligent boy of 13, talked easily with a student about his interests and his disease. He knew other boys with muscular dystrophy whose condition had deteriorated and they had died. Finally he asked 'Will it kill me?'

In the seminar, the student asked 'What do you say?'

Tutorial example 4

Sometimes different groups discussed the same child.

One student was with a four-year-old boy who was suffering from a chronic and potentially fatal disease. Staff were finding him difficult and irritating to manage. On this particular occasion he kept asking the nurses where his mother was. He was told she had just gone down the corridor and would be back soon. In fact, the staff knew she had gone shopping and would be away for some time. On her return the mother gave the boy the same explanation as the staff. She then began showing the staff the things she had bought, talking about them and her trip whilst standing at the foot of the child's bed.

In the next group of students, one described a contact she had with the mother. Whilst she was sitting writing some notes, the boy's mother began a conversation with her. Another patient's mother came up and started talking about something completely different with the first mother. No attempt was made to include the student or to continue or complete the original conversation. The student felt she was being treated as if she was not there and she described the confusion and feeling of impotence this created in her.

In the first of these seminars we discussed the problems for the child in coping with being told lies and then having this compounded by hearing the truth being told in front of him as if he was not there. We discussed the possible implications of this in relation to his ability to trust adults and the relationship to his difficult behaviour. This led to different students giving different parts of the history of the impact of this boy's illness on the whole family. The mother had been told that her son was going to die during the first acute episode of the illness two years previously. She had been able to tell one member of staff that in one way her son had died for her then. Unfortunately she had not been able to accept any more personal support and referral to the child psychiatric team had been turned down. I suggested that this mother was behaving towards the child in part as if he was dead and went on to the issue of the staff responding in the same way. Possible causes of this such as the difficult emotions aroused by working with chronically ill and dying children were then touched upon.

With the second group, having discussed the student's experience and something of the child's illness, I related the information from the previous seminar. I juxtaposed the position of the child in the first incident and the student in the second. I suggested that perhaps the student's experience might give us a better understanding of what the boy was going through. Perhaps his irritating and overbearing behaviour was a way of trying to cope with the emotional turmoil inside himself as a result of this illness and relationship with his mother.

Tutorial example 5

A male student had found himself in an awkward situation.

He had been with a doctor and nurse who were admitting a six-month-old baby to the ward. The baby was suffering from an acute respiratory infection. Her mother was with her but needed to go home to make arrangements for her other children so she had to leave her baby at that point. The doctor had already left and the nurse told the student she had to attend to something else and asked him to stay.

The student said he was not used to babies but finding himself alone with a screaming infant lying in a cot, he had to decide what to do. He sat down next to the cot. He thought the baby was frightened of the situation and of him so he did not try to engage her. He simply observed her through the bars of the cot. She carried on crying but this very gradually began to decrease in intensity. He noticed that she occasionally looked briefly towards him. Eventually her crying stopped.

She then started playing with her toes. After a little while, he touched her fingers and toes; she started playing with his fingers. She then engaged directly with him and he picked her up. The sequence had lasted about 45 minutes. He stayed with her and described her smiling and laughing with him.

The material presented illustrates the powerful challenges and potential of an approach which is based on observation, respectful participation and reflection. Students reported and reflected on having to manage outside their 'comfort zone' in terms of their knowledge, emotional experience and previous experiences of relationships, realising that powerful emotions such as fear, sadness and anger will be evoked. Finding a place for these feelings is essential to avoid disruption of their learning. This requires a learning culture and teaching environment which provides proper respect and support for students in assimilating and processing their new experiences. This, in turn, means teachers engaging in the same processes and having the expectation that their institutions will support such an environment (Tan, Sutton and Dornan 2010).

The students demonstrated respect for the children and acute awareness of the possibility of themselves being a threatening presence (*Tutorial examples 2 and 5*). What they were not so aware of was their potential positive value to the children. I had not originally anticipated this but it became apparent to me from the first tutorial and manifested repeatedly. In *Tutorial example 1*, I suspect the student's spontaneous response and subsequent interactions with this boy may actually have had a therapeutic effect, changing a situation from one of repetition of responses to his defence activity to one in which playfulness could process persecutory experiences. In *Tutorial example 5* I suspect that what could have been a profoundly upsetting experience for the baby became one in which she was able to emerge with an experience of her all-but-overwhelming experiences having been contained. Without setting out to be 'therapeutic' the students had offered something akin to Winnicott's (1971a) descriptions of 'therapeutic consultations'. Indirect benefits also arose from the enhanced understanding of the children and their families which it was possible to feed back to staff involved with their care. This was particularly valuable when it was possible to work as a co-tutor with a paediatrician.

The world of the infant

The infant is born primed for awareness of the presence of another person. This expectation of being in a relationship has been termed *intersubjectivity* (Stern 1985). It sets the stage for a developmental trajectory manifesting the presence or absence of trust and empathy (Trevarthen and Aitken 1994). In psychoanalytic theory this is referred to as *object relations* and various aspects of this have produced intense debate and divergence of views (Likierman 1995).

Klein postulated states of 'paranoid-schizoid functioning' in which 'under-standing' is not a governing principle issue (see e.g. Segal 1988). Processes of projection and identification (Chapter 1) leave room only for two states – 'safety in sameness' in contrast to 'danger in difference'. This is also a world in which there is no sense of absences. If the source of what is desired and experienced as needed is not (objectively) present it is experienced instead as its opposite. It is present but persecuting by withholding what is desired or needed. This is the concept of the *absent object* (O'Shaughnessy 1964). Hunger can be experienced as the presence of a mother who withholds herself and food. With maturation it becomes possible to realise that hunger continues but that there is a not-yet-here-but-wanting-to-feed mother. In states of paranoid schizoid functioning there are no gaps in understanding. Instead these are filled with attributions derived from internal and external cues assimilated into an imaginative life. Recurrence of such experiences later in life gives psychotic experiences as illustrated in *Clinical example 2.4*. For Tony there was no awareness of the IRA being 'recruited' to fill the gap which would otherwise have occurred through not being able to make sense of everything his senses were telling him.

Kleinian theory presents a developmental trajectory of maturation from experience which includes a significant degree of paranoid-schizoid functioning through to an awareness that there are a variety of contribu-tions to experience from the different people involved in relationships. This development includes a sense of having contributed to the state of affairs through one's own wishing and feeling, longing and loving as well as hating and feeling destructive. Klein called this stage *depressive position* (Hinshelwood 1989) which can be confusing since it does not actually refer to depression in the sense of sadness or 'clinical depression'. Winnicott (1963b) took a different position although still building on the underlying framework. He viewed the change as being one of developing a *capacity for concern*. What the baby requires is sufficient experience of their most intense experiences of being contained and harm avoided. Winnicott embodies this by talking of 'holding' rather than containment (see Abram 1996: 183–9). The best foundations for healthier development are laid by the provision of the basics for life along with a necessary and sufficient degree of adaptation and attunement. This ability in the primary carer (mother) and those others available to support her and her baby is crucial in promoting emotional development (Murray and Andrews 2000; Murray et al. 2011).

The philosophical and psychodynamic consideration of trust and primitive states provides a framework to consider how relationships become estab-lished and used to promote 'understanding' in its fullest sense. Knowing our place as clinicians in people's lives involves applying our knowledge and training in the service of our patients. In doing this we have to ensure that our personal interests – our inquisitiveness, our need to learn, our need to earn a living, our wish to be recognised by others – are neither obtrusive nor intrusive.

Making things add up in relationships

Some years ago I was watching a sports programme which was part of the coverage of Wimbledon tennis tournament. The presenters were discussing the different practice and expectations of commentators. They illustrated this by showing two commentators watching and listening to a BBC broadcast and then discussing it. The excerpt showed the two leading players involved in an exhilarating rally. It seemed impossible that either should have been able to return the ball let alone produce a further challenge to the protagonist. This was accompanied by the gasps of the spectators and the silence of the commentators. At the end, one of the commentators simply let out an exclamation of admiration and appreciation. The observing commentators simply could not understand the sound of silence.

Winnicott was interested in the processes of people being able to experience what is happening without needing to feel a sense of agency in the immediate situation and in being able to resist any impulse unhelpfully to make themselves agents. He was a master of the enigmatic aphorism and summed up the importance of this ability as 'after being – doing and being done to. But first, being' (Winnicott 1971a: 85).

Appreciating our place in other people's lives is a fundamental indicator of social development. Our place may be in deciding to be present or absent, to make things happen or not to make things happen. By extension, Winnicott was also interested in how it is possible to be with another person without necessarily being observably, actively engaged with that person. He called this 'the capacity to be alone' (Winnicott 1958: 30). There is a paradox in this in that 'this experience is that of being alone, as an infant and small child, in the presence of mother'. Thus the basis of the capacity to be alone is a paradox; it is the experience of being alone while someone is present. The essential ingredient is the capacity to act without the need to involve the other person in doing something or to provoke an experience in the other – making her feel she has been 'done-to' – in order to carry on with the activity. This indicates a degree of equanimity in terms of there being neither conscious nor unconscious pressures from either person: it is a state in which the processes of projective identification are not called upon.

The sports commentators who were observing their colleagues did not appear to have attained this 'capacity to be alone'. Or perhaps it would be fairer to say that they had not been able to maintain it. They were driven by a need to feel they were creating the viewers' experience. The BBC commentators were able to be there, ready to enhance the experience but able to be present alongside others as co-observers. The observing commentators, driven by the imperative 'Don't just *sit* there, *do* something!', were not able to follow a different imperative 'Don't just *do* something, *sit* there!' The observing commentators might have argued that their employers required them to 'do' something, and that the action of their colleagues would have been a 'breach of contract'. But their need (for employment in a culture which wants immediate, immediately identifiable impact) takes precedence over serving to enhance experience.

Developing an ability to manage what happens inside us as practitioners in observing our patients is essential. Knowing when action is required and knowing when 'externalising' (i.e. observable activity) is not required both require mental activity. Deciding which is required and in what balance at which time can come easily to some people and less easily to others; it is a factor in all practice with children and their carers. It becomes particularly critical in working with mothers and babies and in general when using psychoanalytic approaches. For this reason, infant observation is a requirement in psychoanalytic psychotherapy trainings and can be beneficial for all work with children (Miller et al. 1989).

Contending with the relationships between other people and finding one's place with them includes finding oneself as an observer to their relationship. Stern (1990) pointed out how three-person relationships actually involve six relationships, If we consider three people, A, B and C, then we have relationships of A to B, B to C and C to A (Figure 4a). In addition we have A in relation to B's relationship with C (Figure 4b) plus the same for the other pairings. So, any group of three people automatically involves at least six relationships (Figure 4c).[5]

The recurrent theme is that by placing ourselves in professional roles we inevitably put ourselves in situations of increasing relational complexity. We create the possibility of the emergence of feelings, thoughts and less easily identifiable experiences which must be managed. Failure to do so may have serious consequences for our patients and ourselves. In addition to the countertransference issues described in Chapter 1 we have to develop the ability to manage ourselves in relation to the relationships between other people.

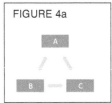

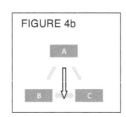

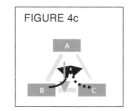

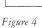
Figure 4

Mothers and babies

In the ordinary course of events, at the centre of the process of birth and the puerperium are two people who are adjusting to a massive reorientation and reorganisation. During pregnancy a mother has been able to do all her baby needed simply by looking after herself properly but now she has to apply herself differently to her baby's needs. Becoming established together requires confidence that she and her baby are suitably equipped to survive and thrive and in her own ability to provide what is needed for their 'equipment' to function. The experience can be a pleasure and a pain: the quality and intensity of experience, unique. Awareness of what she can now do for her baby opens the way to realising and learning more about her own abilities. She can also be faced with an emergence of fears that she may not have it in herself to do what is needed. Accompanying this may be the stirring up of conscious or unconscious fears that she will do harm. Winnicott (1956a) described this period as *primary maternal preoccupation.* The mother's needs and the baby's needs are so intimately linked that they are inseparable to the extent that 'There is no such thing as a baby ... if you set out to describe a baby, you will find you are describing a *baby and someone.* A baby cannot exist alone, but is essentially part of a relationship' (Winnicott 1964: 88).

As clinicians our first responsibility is to respect this by being available to participate if needed and to ensure we do this in the least intrusive and obtrusive way possible. Only in situations of particular need, for example illness in mother or baby, should there be need to come between them. When it is necessary, any interventions should be mediated as far as possible through those who are and will continue to be in the most important relationships, for example fathers, extended family.

Beyond staying alive and in reasonable health, perhaps the most important thing a mother can do for her baby is feed her. The evidence is that the benefits to be gained from breastfeeding in terms of physical health in the short term and through life far outweigh those of artificial substitutes. Yet in the UK breastfeeding rates remain poor.[6]

Where recommendations exist relating to other areas of child health, my experience is that practitioners appear to feel free to be vociferous, and even strident, in their views and efforts to see that they are adhered to, for example parents who decide not to immunise their child may be openly criticised. Yet the growth-promoting and health-providing benefits of breast milk over artificial formula feeds do not appear to produce an equivalent response. The supply of a mother's milk is responsive in part to her baby's needs. If an artificial mechanism was found for replicating this would there be any hesitation in recommending it over currently available alternatives? This is a highly complex area but in the present context I want to consider if psychodynamic factors may affect whether health practitioners robustly apply evidence-based recommendations.[7]

There is a proper concern for mothers who might not be able to breastfeed for any reason and full and proper account needs to be taken of their position. But these women are not so numerous as to govern general policies rather than ensuring the provision of high-quality, individualised care. Paternalistic health practices have been challenged and the importance of personal autonomy and choice has come more to the fore. But personal autonomy and choice do not necessarily make good bedfellows with parenthood – particularly not where the care of babies and young children are concerned. In fact, the ways in which the ordinarily devoted parents' welfare and sense of well-being are dependent on their child's welfare cannot be underestimated. Winnicott (1956a: 308) again captures this: 'when we are able to help parents to help their children we do in fact help them about themselves'.

The factors involved generate heated debate despite the scientific evidence. The factors influencing breastfeeding being chosen and supported are multiple (Raphael-Leff 1991: 551). In clinical practice, advocating it wholeheartedly may be inhibited by professionals recognising that their training is insufficient for the task or that the opportunities to fulfil the role adequately are limited by other demands. However, faint praise or reluctance to be an advocate may tip the balance and rob a mother and baby of something beneficial.

Where infant feeding is concerned, I have observed many professionals switch into a different mode, sharing either that they did not breastfeed or that they found it difficult. My impression is that this happens more readily than in other areas of practice. As a man I am freed from having any personal experience of being a breastfeeding mother. But if I had that experience would I use it explicitly with reference to it being what happened to me and how I handled it? Sharing may be an enlightened attempt to correct perceived power imbalances and to enhance a lay-mother's self-esteem; sharing a difficulty in order to demonstrate that clinical expertise does not confer expertise in personal life. But a problem shared is not necessarily a problem halved. It may undermine recognition that this mother does have it in her or that very different contingencies apply to the situation. It offers a spurious authority reminiscent of the UK government minister who fed his child beef to prove that there was no potential problem of infection with vCJD.

Brandell (1992: 35–44) highlighted how a professional's *identification with the patient* may come into play unhelpfully and how it needs to be distinguished from what can properly be attributed to the patient's transference or projective processes. In psychoanalytic theory acknowledgement or denial of difference plays a crucial role (see for example Segal 1988); the corollary is that unconscious envy can be a particularly powerful force in the countertransference. It can be a manifestation of deprivations, of awareness of dependence on what others possess and one's dependence on them. It can stem from longings and resonances with good experiences in the past that cannot be regained, of Paradise lost. Identificatory processes pre-empt acceptance of difference. They may feel like the forging of a respectful partnership but rather than respecting autonomy it may unwittingly undermine it. They 'manage' something in the immediate situation and deal with the unprocessed and unconscious experiences which the practitioner brings. The patient looks after the professional.

The feelings evoked in being with a mother and baby can lead to an unconscious enactment of envy which manifests as a need to be a prime actor in feeding the baby rather than a facilitating influence. Inability to tolerate the pain or frustrations that may be experienced by mother or baby may lead to premature interventions in feeding, undermining the potential of the relationship between mother and baby to be realised. A fathers' involvement in the care of their baby has to take account of this: being a father should not be equated with being simply interchangeable with the mother and any wish to be involved in feeding should not come in the way of what the baby needs. He has a key role as the first representative of the persistence of the outside world beyond the foundation relationship (eee for example Abram 1996: 169–71). Neither should fathers be used simply as a repository for projections of envy – assuming they will feel pushed out or envious rather than accepting their experience of a multitude of emotions as they play their part in the new relationships that are forming.

For all these reasons many organisations involved in training those who may be involved with new babies and their mothers in their feeding relationship are required to go through a process of 'debriefing' their own experiences and being able to demonstrate they have assimilated them in a way that will not intrude into their patients' and clients' lives.

When special care is needed

The range of conditions which would previously have been incompatible with life in newborn infants but which can now be treated has risen enormously. Care of premature babies has expanded to such an extent that new challenges are faced in medical ethics and law in deciding when the rights of 'personhood' are confirmed. With these new advances come new challenges to parents and professionals to understand not only their use and applications but also to contend with the experience of them being applied. McFadyen (1994) has written about the care and development of relationships of babies admitted to medical special care bay units and neonatal intensive care units. What follows is an account of my work with some child psychiatrist colleagues, who were at the time nearing the end of their specialist training, in a related type of unit, a surgical special care baby unit (Surgical SCBU).

Developing relationships: the value of research in child psychiatric liaison

The Surgical SCBU in St Mary's Hospital, Manchester, recognised very early in its establishment the importance of an holistic approach to the families of infants admitted to their unit. The staff were particularly concerned about the long-term adjustments of the families and the babies. And this led to the establishment of *family care nurses*. These posts were at senior level and served to bridge the gap between hospital and home, assisting parents in the sometimes highly complicated tasks involved in the care of their babies. I received a request from the unit for some teaching about the experiences of parents whose babies were on the unit over a long period of time. I did not have specific experience in this arena but what was as important in deciding what to do was the fact that the request for teaching could be understood as a referral for help with a 'systemic symptom'. The information I was given indicated that this had arisen as a new area of concern because some compli- cated situations had arisen. I arranged a process of initial 'consultation to the system' rather than a simple teaching exercise.[8] I arranged a series of meetings with nursing staff to better understand their work and the various issues arising from this. I also met one of the mothers; this was arranged on the basis of asking for her assistance in helping us understand more about the issues for parents when their child is on the unit for a long time. The meetings highlighted four particular areas:

1 Communication problems between staff within the same discipline, between staff of different disciplines and between staff and parents. Added to this were complexities consequent upon the various permutations, for example information communicated to a parent by a doctor might not be given to nursing staff directly from the doctor but rather by the parent on the basis of the parents' understanding and/or misunderstanding.
2 Some babies' problems altered from being those of acute surgical/technical care through to becoming 'long-term' nursing and infant care without the baby being well enough to be discharged. At this point there was a clear change in relationships between parents and nursing staff. During the acute stage the primary influence on the nurse–parent relationship was in terms of technical expertise and, in this respect, nurses were experienced as being more or less interchangeable. However, as the babies became 'long term', the individual personalities of the parents and staff were more significant for the relationship: the 'fit' was more important. The result was that clear preferences would arise in relationships and, as a consequence, the potential for rivalries and conflicts.
3 The powerful forces at play in (1) and (2) in the context of infants with such serious or even life-threatening illnesses created a situation in which the conflicts were more likely to be experienced or enacted.
4 The depth of concern and thought about the issues of relationships for babies and their parents was impressive; the request for child psychiatric involvement was a demonstration of this.

My preferred response would have been to offer ongoing consultation to the staff group; however, child psychiatric resources did not allow this possibility.

Instead I wrote an open letter to the staff describing my observations as outlined above. There remained the opportunity for any specific family who felt they needed child psychiatric assessment to be referred through the usual routes.

Through learning we teach

An opportunity subsequently arose for a period of detailed work with the Surgical SCBU through a fortunate combination of events. The unit identified a further area of specified need. Simultaneously two trainees with appropriate sub-specialist experience and allocated time for clinical research developed an interest in this area. Below they describe finding themselves in a new clinical world.

Dr Smith

As a senior trainee on the ward round in the paediatric medical ward I expressed interest in a baby, Josh, aged two months whose mother was objecting to the use of a dummy/pacifier in her care. Nurses explained that Josh had had surgery to his throat and been tube fed. They felt that the dummy would help him to learn to suck. I spent time with the mother and realised the impact of her son's feeding difficulty upon their relationship. We agreed to keep in contact. Over the four months that followed I had eight meetings with Josh and his mother. He had a complicated surgical course and I found myself drawn into my first conversation with the surgeon and the surgical nurses about the impact of a feeding problem on a developing mother–child relationship.

In this time with Josh and his mother I had to come to terms with the intrusive presence of the monitors. Josh had frequent respiratory arrests. (I was greatly relieved that he never stopped breathing during my sessions.) His mother talked with me about her feelings for the baby and how the technology of the monitor had a particular role in her awareness of her baby.

This close encounter with a mother and baby in crisis was the beginning of my relationship with the neonatal surgical team. I was both interested as a doctor and a psychiatrist and at the same time shocked by the experience. As the mother became an expert about her baby's condition, I too learnt from her. As a child psychiatrist I felt perplexed by the extensive network of highly skilled people and expensive machinery surrounding a developing mother–child relationship. I was unsure of my role and with my colleagues decided to capitalise on a model of liaison developed in Manchester by Professor Elena Garralda which forges links through joint research into the

---

psychological experience of patients and families. This made sense in a psychoanalytic model; research is seen as seeking understanding within a relationship with paediatric staff. More pragmatically it offered a route forward as time for research could be protected from clinical demands.

Dr Jones, a fellow trainee, joined us in an embryonic research group. Her interest in mothers and babies establishing their relationship had also emerged from direct clinical work with a mother and her seriously ill baby:

'Over the course of about a year I had to work out where I fitted into a new way of working in parent-infant therapy. At the same time I had to contend with my feelings of not knowing about babies and their illnesses.'

We tentatively approached the surgeons with a plan for research with the aim of finding out how a child psychiatrist can contribute to the assessment and care of newborns with congenital abnormalities which can be treated by surgery. The surgical team were keen to establish this. It was agreed that in selected cases where they felt there would be benefit, mothers would be offered a consultation with a psychiatrist. They thought this would help us to establish our role in the unit and to develop our ideas for research.

The task of planning our involvement was a consultative exercise in itself. Dr Smith and Dr Jones met with the surgeons and with the nurses several times during day and night shifts to discuss with them what we hoped to do and to seek their views. This began the establishment of a working relationship. It enabled our role to be distinguished from that of the social worker who potentially could have become involved with any of the babies. Dr Jones was struck by the parallels between her experience of learning about parent–infant therapy and the emerging clinical research process:

'In the same way, in approaching this project we were needing to learn how to fit into this strange new world that we had discovered. We quickly become aware that the surgeons and the nurses had their own separate areas of expertise, in the theatre and at the cot. But we did not know where our expertise might lie.'

At first we were surprised in our conversations with the surgeons at the artfulness and creativity that went into the operations. Operations were done that were not described in any textbook but were an individualised response to a particular baby's anatomy. We had not realised how similar surgery could be to psychiatry in having to deal with uncertainty and not-knowing. Our initial feelings of ignorance carried with them anxiety which decreased as our questions were responded to thoughtfully and respectfully. It appeared to be a relief to the staff that questions could be asked and answers sought. Thus it became a shared endeavour of seeking to know what it was really like for these parents and their babies on the unit and if child psychiatrists could be useful to them.

The Surgical SCBU was like a world in itself, perched, constantly lit, atop the hospital tower. Nurses sometimes felt they were not part of the normal hospital life, forgotten and not noticed even though the lights were always on. There was a powerful sense of paradox of being isolated yet on display. The nurses echoed the feeling expressed by one mother about her baby's simultaneous isolation and public display in his incubator. This mother was able to recognise that her feeling was not only what she thought her baby would be experiencing. It was her own experience of being with her baby, at times with him but at others isolated from him in the presence of other people. Whatever she did it could be viewed by other people.

Below are some representative comments from consultations with mothers:

> 'They took me down to the SCBU... It was shattering. She was in an incubator, I was in a wheelchair... I couldn't touch her... I was totally drained. He had things sticking out all over: monitors; a tube up his nose ... mucus coming out of everywhere – mouth, nose. I couldn't believe that that was mine.'
>
> 'He just looked at me and I loved him. I just wanted to forget that this was happening.'
>
> 'I thought "it's a bad dream, someone's going to wake me up". She just didn't look normal ... Normal babies, they look contented or cry. She just laid there.'
>
> 'I only saw him once before he was taken to St Mary's. I only held him once. I didn't have energy for a proper cuddle. All this equipment everywhere. Nothing about him looked right ... it was terrifying.'
>
> 'It just didn't seem like she was mine. Everything was unreal. Where was this perfect baby we'd expected ... I had this tiny thing that didn't look very well ... I suppose without realising it I switched myself off from the baby...'

We came to understand how the issue of display and intrusion were inter-linked. For the nurses our presence was another form of people being put on display. At first some had been suspicious of what child psychiatrists may be doing on the unit – one nurse asked if we were analysing them. We learnt a lot from informal conversations with nurses and parents, often 'over the cot'.

Dr Jones describes a specific episode:

On one occasion I watched a baby having his nasal passages sucked out by a nurse using a plastic tube and a suction pump. The baby was squirming and his mother who was watching closely looked uncomfortable. But the nurse handled the procedure in a professional way – without looking uncomfortable and being useful and efficient.

The procedure although minor and routine was invasive for the baby. I was aware that I was feeling invasive just by being there and witnessing this activity and the mother's distress. This reminded me that I could indeed be invasive for the mothers by my physical presence. I could come to see them on the ward whenever I wanted to but the ward became their home – several mothers had stated that home is where their baby is. I realised I needed to learn to allow the mothers to *not* want to see me sometimes.

The problem of ensuring good communication was one with which we could help:

One mother was very anxious that her baby was not putting on weight. She thought he may have malabsorption like her husband's sister. She had tried to ask the surgeon if he would transfer the baby's care to a physician. She thought that would enable the baby to have tests or treatment that he had not had. However the surgeon did not think that was needed and the mother's anxiety remained unresolved.

The nurses saw this as the mother having had an opportunity to talk with the surgeon, but for some reason, not wanting to listen to him. The nurses were feeling inhibited about discussing the issue further with her because they in turn were anxious about an aspect of her mothering that they had observed. They thought that the mother was interpreting her infant's difficulty in feeding as wilfulness or naughtiness. Mother would tell her baby not to be naughty when he had difficulty feeding, and the infant was described as 'good' by both nurses and mother when he was feeding well. Thus a moral dimension had been imposed and the infant was presumed to have some self-will in this domain.

When I went to meet with the mother, she seemed relieved to talk and said almost immediately that she was worried because the nurses were calling her baby naughty. She said she realised that he was not being either naughty or good, and it was annoying her that the nurses were making such presumptions. The issue therefore raised itself naturally. She went on to explain and think about her feelings that the surgeon was being over-possessive of her baby.

It was as if the surgeon did indeed have ownership of the baby. He had maintained his life and the mother had 'merely' brought the baby into the world. Her fear of the surgeon's perceived wish to possess the baby prevented her from pressing her point and she had remained anxious and dissatisfied. But she had been unable to say all this to the staff; she explained to me that she did not want to be critical when they had done so much to help. This cleared the air for discussions and the reasons for misunderstandings and difficulties in relationships were themselves understood. Trust and confidence were restored.

This situation also brought out the appreciation of infants' individual characters and how far they were recognised as individuals by the nurses. We saw that with the key nurse system as far as possible the babies and their nurses know each other. Being a key nurse gave permission for an individualised concern for the babies. It also led us to consider the different aspects of the nursing role – one aspect akin to a 'primary maternal preoccupation' (Winnicott 1956a), the other a 'primary surgical preoccupation'.

Concern for the individual was an area that we thought we would like to consider in detail in the interviews with the mother. We were interested in how her concern for her baby's individual experience was manifest. We thought it would be reflected in the current state of the mother's mental organisation and her thoughts and feelings regarding attachment. For example, a mother said that when her baby looked at her for the first time she knew that he was telling her that he wanted to be held and cuddled. She was able to do what she could for him by stroking the back of his head and said that when she did that he knew he was being cared for.

The full complexity of what could happen was emphasised in the situation of a mother who had had a multiple birth: two of the babies were very seriously ill and had to remain in hospital while the others were able to go home.

Dr Jones

Six months after delivery one baby was well enough to go home to be with the rest of the family. The nurses then became worried because mother did not seem to spend much time on the ward and was arriving later and later.

Mother explained to me that she did not feel right when she was away from home because she missed the babies who were at home so much. She did not feel right when she was at home either, because she missed the baby that was in hospital.

For the next meeting, Mother brought in a photograph of the babies who were at home. She stood it beside the baby in hospital while we talked. She said that for the first time she had all her babies in her mind together. She was able to describe her feelings of love for her ill daughter, how beautiful she was, how she enjoyed touching her and looking into her eyes, how she missed her when she was not there and how she felt relieved and comforted to see her.

The conflict between fear of isolation and freedom from intrusion is profoundly complicated. There seemed to be a particular value in our role as people who came into and left this mind-boggling world of lights and sounds and vulnerability but who were also accepted as a non-intrusive presence. Being this 'someone else' for mothers did seem to facilitate them in finding it possible to be alone and establish themselves more with their babies. Usually this process of getting started together is an intimate partnership between 'being with' and 'doing to': doing can make easier the process of being with when it might otherwise become too difficult. They had to be able to tolerate other people doing things to their baby and their babies' consequent distress. These mothers had to find a way of containing their impulses for action in the face of not being able to do the usual things for their babies. They had to learn about their babies in the context of their baby's 'not-doing' and mutual responsiveness not being possible in the usual way.

Dr Jones

I watched a mother struggling to play with her month old and very ill baby who was unable to respond. It is very hard to get the balance right between being too stimulating and not being stimulating enough. In that case, it was frustratingly impossible for the mother to enable normal development to take place in the abnormal environment. She expressed the conflict between her longing for escape from that environment and her baby's dependency on it: she wished she could steal her baby away with her in her shopping bag – but she knew if she did he would die.

The observations here have come out of using a model based in a particular form of participant observation. It attends very carefully to maintaining awareness of the different clinical roles and the place of being authorised to observe and offer a commentary. We helped parents to understand their feelings or actions and help them to regain a sense of coherence which facilitated their relationship with their infant. We assisted staff to understand why a particular parent is feeling or behaving in a certain way. In addition to the work with mothers, individual nurses discussed issues that concerned them such as the need for privacy in bereavement and the difficulty of accepting death. We were able to go beyond the 'primary surgical preoccupation', helping nurses and mothers in understanding their role and what they can do.

Summary and conclusions

Entering the world of clinical practice is a developmental milestone accompanied by events and processes building on previous qualities and learning and opening up new possibilities of what we can do and what can happen to us in this process. Becoming part of other people's lives through our professional role opens us up to things about ourselves as well as about those other people who look to us at particular times of need. This is never more so than at the start of life when mothers and babies are becoming established together. It requires a particular sensitivity to the impact we may have on others and the impact they have upon us. A fundamental respect for autonomy, dependence and interdependence combined with an openness to learning provides a sound base for the emergence of trustworthiness and for our patients, their parents and colleagues to have confidence in us. Such trustworthiness is the platform from which good clinical practice and research can emerge.

4

STEPPING INTO THE UNKNOWN

If you have men who will only come if they know there is a good road, I don't want them. I want men who will come if there is no road at all.[1]

Illness places us in the position of relying on people who do routinely what is in everyday life extraordinary. Expecting or knowing that they have dealt with such situations before can be immensely reassuring. To have a sense of our lack of uniqueness in our predicament may be consoling. But if we feel that our individuality has not been acknowledged we may be left feeling badly treated.

Uncharted territory

As practitioners we have to be able to see similarities and define differences, both in the biomedical and in the psychosocial sphere. We need to be able to recognise when we are in the area of unknowns, beyond the routine, uncommon or rare, into the unique. When this applies we have to assess how well-equipped we are to proceed or whether someone else can best serve the patient. Extending the boundaries of what is possible brings with it the possibility of unexpected biomedical consequences: it also brings with it the unknown qualities or quantities of life for those people who will be living with the consequences.

Clinical example 4.1(a)

The Surgical Special Care Baby Unit requested my input with the parents of a child born with severe complex anatomical abnormalities of the lower abdomen.[2] The message explained that immediate decisions needed to be made and that there would be long-term issues involving further surgical interventions.

When I returned the call, by chance, the surgeon himself answered. He explained that the child's problems included genital abnormalities of a severity which raised the issue of gender assignment. The received wisdom was that in children with XY chromosomes the children

---

should be 'assigned' as female through surgical procedures. The basis for this was that it would provide for a more ordinary external genital appearance and the provision of a vagina although no other female organs could be constructed.[3] He further explained that he found it very difficult to know what to do since his experience was that text books could be wrong and in such rare conditions there was no robust evidence for the recommendations made.

His most immediate dilemma was to decide how he could advise the parents. There were anatomical and hormonal considerations some aspects of which derived from current knowledge but other aspects took him into unknown territory. He was simultaneously considering the predicament of the child and his parents, both in terms of the immediate trauma and the future implications whichever course of action was taken. He described various contingencies he needed to hold in mind. He would not have enough details about the child's condition until he was carrying out the operation, identifying the anatomical structures and their state of development and relationship to each other through the process of dissection.

Listening to his description, the enormity of what he was grappling with was clear. My only specific comments related to my view of the need to hold fully in mind that the child was his patient, the parents were not. This was not said to diminish their experience or rights, but to keep in mind the axiom 'if we help a parent parent, we help a parent'.

The surgeon was able to formulate what he could describe to the parents. He could give a reasonable description of what possibilities may arise but he was not in a position to describe the probabilities of different constellations occurring. The corollary was that there was an enormous range of prognoses, remarkable for their uncertainties rather than any indications of what was more or less likely. He could only give them the facts and ask for their permission to make judgements in the process of the operation.

The surgeon's dilemmas were highly complex not only technically but ethically. In seeking to provide information what he had to present was uncertainty and lack of knowledge in conjunction with his recognised knowledge and technical proficiency. In seeking the parents' assent to proceed along certain lines, the term 'informed consent' does not seem to capture the extent to which it is a process of seeking to become better informed, in another person's judgement, despite their uncertainty and tolerating 'not-knowing'. All that can be aspired to and expected is that any course of action is well-reasoned and balances risks and benefits. In conjunction with this is an expectation that all possible steps will be taken to respond to what follows, particularly any untoward effects, in a humane way.

Actions need to be considered not only in terms of the direct consequences but also in terms of the implications and further obligations that may arise. The situation cannot be understood simply as being the negotiations between a clinician and the parents on behalf of their child. There are implications far beyond their combined abilities and commitment. The intricacies extend beyond the scope of this present exposition, but the processes involved rely on clarity of the bounds of personal, professional and organisational autonomy and authority: for all parties the challenges of trusting one's own judgement and motivation and those of others' can be considerable.

These ethical considerations are not strictly the realm of expertise of child psychiatry. But ethical analysis does need to be informed by an understanding of the psychological implications of practice. My psychiatric contribution in this immediate situation was best understood in terms of holding in mind the psychological complexity and turbulence for all parties. In being a receptacle for these, in partnership with the surgeon, his thinking could be freed from some of the disruptive effects of feeling solely responsible.

Clinical example 4.1(b)

Some years later Dennis was referred for a second opinion by a colleague who knew that I had seen a number of children with unusual sexual and genital development. Dennis and his parents had experienced a highly complicated and rocky journey. He had required prolonged hospital care with repeated episodes of life-threatening illness. He had eventually been able to live outside hospital but he could not be cared for in a family setting. When referred he was being looked after on his own by a team of experienced child care staff who were providing what I have come to think of as a sort of social, emotional and educational 'incubator'.

I arranged to see him with a senior member of the care staff whom it was felt he could most trust. From the information already available, it sounded likely that Dennis would find attendance difficult and was unlikely to be able to tolerate an individual consultation. In addition, the immediate care situation was proving so difficult that I felt a participatory consultative process with the staff was more likely to provide 'First Aid', offering both containment and an opportunity for Dennis and his carer to find out about me and how I would approach the situation.

It was a challenging consultation for all three of us but Dennis was able to engage with me with the help of his carer who was also able to explain in Dennis's presence what some of the difficulties were. Dennis did not find this easy but was able to tolerate it with his carer's help.

In considering the specific involvement of health care professionals an interesting dynamic emerged. Dennis had very different views and feelings about medical and nursing staff. Nurses were safer and doctors more threatening. I explored this further and what Dennis was able to explain was that it was because the doctors had literally been inside him, they knew him inside and out. But from his point of view the nurses had not seen or been inside him. The feelings which arose in him from this were at times unmanageable. I reflected this back to him in terms of how being known very well could feel like being known **too** well: he agreed that it could feel this way even though he also realised he needed to be understood.

Dennis had been told that I was part of the clinical team involved just after his birth and this was interesting for him. I also emphasised that I was a doctor and that this might be significant in terms of his feelings about me in view of what he had said about doctors. My responses to him had also been informed by experience of work with children where genital development did not occur normally but I did not make this explicit.

Dennis immediately takes us into the fundamental realm of psychosomatic relations. The skin does literally define us and it is within this container that our sense of personal identity emerges.[5] What also facilitates this individuation, and is ultimately required for a mature sense of individual identity, separate from other people, is the realisation that there can be parts of the self which another person cannot know. It became ever clearer how profound the challenges were for Dennis in this respect. He was reliant on being known extremely well but at times this felt too much for him: he felt intruded upon and persecuted by it. This was exemplified by his subsequent persistent, intense ambivalence about me. I was never sure whether or not my comments to him in that first consultation had unwittingly fuelled this or if it was inevitable. Although they had seemed accurate, appropriate and 'modulating' in the terms described in Chapters 1 and 2, my reflections back to him about being known inside and out may have been premature. He needed to know simultaneously that I could not know or understand things about him.

Clinical example 4.1(c)

I obtained detailed descriptions of Dennis's day-to-day activities and events in his life. Of particular concern were repeated episodes of extreme outbursts of violent behaviour (challenging behaviour) after which Dennis would be physically exhausted and often apologetic when he had recovered. Staff attempted to manage and alter these through a behavioural modification approach of seeking to reinforce 'positive' behaviour and avoid reinforcement of 'negative'. His behaviour was seen as manipulative in the sense of 'If he doesn't get his own way he has a tantrum'.

I felt that I needed to challenge this idea that these episodes were 'wilful', 'controlled behaviour'. However, I was also very conscious of how easily staff might view this as dismissive of the seriousness of the actual events and the determination with which they persisted in their efforts to ensure the safety of all concerned. I offered alternative explanations such as those derived from the original descriptions of children separated from their parents (Robertson and Robertson 1989) and Attachment Theory (see Bowlby 1977).

I also focused very carefully on the impact on the staff through these events and the way they were left feeling when an episode came to an end. They felt physically exhausted and mentally drained. I presented a formulation of this in terms of processes of projective identification and failure of defence mechanisms. Rather than his behaviour being seen as a mechanism to manipulate others and exploit situations, I presented it as defensive processes beyond his control which came into action in response to an internal state of extreme threat.[6] I suggested that their feelings could inform us about Dennis's experiences.

A key additional aspect of all this was the extreme challenge the episodes presented to the staff in managing themselves with him. In discussions with the senior managers involved, I explained that the intensity was such that even extremely experienced staff might find themselves feeling at a loss as to what to do, overwhelmed, and then act uncharacteristically. The risk of loss of impulse control needed to be acknowledged and taken into account in the assessment of the risks for all parties if a proper framework to support the staff in the care of Dennis was to be put in place.

Despite the very different theoretical foundations from which the staff and I were developing our formulations and the different contributions we could make, my approach ultimately provided a solid basis for partnership in providing a care environment for Dennis. Ensuring sufficient attention was paid to the impact of caring for him upon the staff (in both acute situations and in the long term) was not to set their needs against his but to describe what was necessary and sufficient to enable them to fulfil their roles. Despite even extensive experience and the best will in the world, the potential for someone to act 'unprofessionally' was such that staff needed exceptional consideration and acceptance. This was not to license bad practice or malpractice but to demonstrate awareness of the need Dennis had for a total environment which promoted true empathy and trust.

Most clinical practice does not deal with extremely unusual conditions. A doctor reading a referral letter may have read similar descriptions many times before, but he still needs to be ready for the uniqueness of each person's experience and his own responses to this. There is a great difference between a doctor who has seen a condition 100 times and a doctor who has really met 100 people with that condition.

Recovering ground

For any new patient and her carers, entering the clinic or hospital is a step into the unknown. However, alongside awareness of the novelty, they may have preformed expectations based on previous experiences. Some of these may be conscious and readily identifiable – the child who has had immunisations fearing that we are going to stick a needle into her; the parents who were seen by a child psychiatrist as a child and who expect the same general approach to their child and themselves. Past experience may also operate at an unconscious level, directly affecting immediate reactions in a way that might very readily be understandable if the previous experience is identified, for example a parent's forgotten traumatic childhood experience of hospitals creating anxiety when taking her child to hospital. Other unconscious influences may become understandable through the concept of transference.

The paradox of transference is that even if the relationship with this new doctor is recognisably new, it is not new. It is an old script looking for a new actor in one of the roles. If we manage the countertransference correctly, we can prevent the old story simply being re-told. In Chapter 1, I described how I 'acted out in the countertransference' (*Clinical Example 1.2*). I was able to re-establish the process of parent–infant therapy with Mrs T and her daughter through realising and acknowledging my mistake. The fuller story gives more indications of how important this was.

Clinical example 4.2(a)

An assistant paediatrician asked me to see Mrs T and her 15-month-old child because of serious difficulties in their relationship. They were attending the paediatric clinic as a follow-up to neonatal problems. I arranged for the initial appointment to be conducted jointly with the paediatrician as I thought this was likely to assist assessment

---

and ensure good communication. During the consultation it became clear that Mrs T had significant conflicts about attending the clinic. I addressed this explicitly. At the end of the consultation I told her I thought the department could be of use to her and her daughter but that I thought she needed time to decide what she wanted to do. The arrangement was that she could contact me if she wished to arrange another appointment.

I did not hear anything for six months but then Mrs T phoned to ask for another appointment. This was the beginning of an extended contact. I saw her and her daughter, Lisa, during the initial phase of therapy.

Asking for help with the problems she and Lisa were having had been very difficult. She had attended out of desperation rather than from expectation of any good coming from it. However, gradually she felt able to trust me more and feel there was realistic hope of things getting better. After a few sessions, she began to tell me about her own severe problems in adolescence. This arose because I had noted a particular pattern in the description of feeding difficulties in the first few months. These made me wonder if Mrs T had had eating difficulties herself so I asked her about this. I was taken aback by her response.

She replied 'My mother told me not to tell you.'

Mrs T had had inpatient psychiatric treatment in late adolescence because of an eating disorder. She described having battles with staff and her parents. She told me that her parents had lied to staff at times. When she protested about this she was never believed: her protestations were seen as further evidence of her disorder.

The nature of Mrs T's adolescent difficulties and their effect on parenting were topics in which I had a special interest. As the parent–infant therapy became more robustly established, I mistakenly asked about having access to her psychiatric records.

When I next saw her, I told her that I had not requested the notes because I thought I had made a mistake in asking and I apologised. I explained why I thought I had been wrong. Mrs T told me that although she had felt free in giving consent, she had felt extremely anxious coming for this session. She was worried that I might have seen the notes and changed my view of her. We discussed this further before re-establishing the focus on the relationship between her and Lisa.

During the next period of therapy Lisa's father was able to attend some appointments. Later, it became possible to offer Lisa individual psychotherapy with a colleague. I undertook the continuing work with her parents, principally with the mother, and I also maintained contact with the paediatric staff involved.

As the work progressed, it was apparent that Mrs T had considerable obsessional symptoms in addition to continued conflict about food. Food was also a point of conflict between Mrs T and Lisa. However, improvements did gradually occur. These were underlined by Mrs T one day describing Lisa smearing her chocolate-covered hands over some spotlessly clean kitchen cupboard doors. In relating this she told me, 'I realised that I really wanted to do that!'

Exploration of her childhood experiences provided an understanding of just how important the issue of being believed or disbelieved was. Mrs T described the conflicts there had been between her parents. She remembered times when her father would return home drunk having left her mother dealing with family matters. Her mother had on occasions told her father lies about Mrs T, saying she had been misbehaving while he was out. Her father would physically chastise her despite her protestations: the more she protested, the more she was beaten. He would later beg her forgiveness.

On another occasion she had needed a routine health procedure which required an injection. She had been so terrified that the procedure had had to be postponed. This had earned her a beating with the threat of more if the events were repeated. On the next visit she was meek and compliant despite her terror. What came across most strongly in recounting this was her disbelief that the practitioner, who knew her fairly well, did not comment on the change nor seem to be puzzled by how dramatic it was.

The importance of practitioners maintaining clarity about their role with parents is particularly significant for the work of child mental specialists in considering what it means to 'work with' parents when a child is being treated in individual psychotherapy. Lynette Hughes and I (2005) argued that there are such specific theoretical, technical issues and clinical implications it deserves to be recognised as a specialist area of practice which we called 'the psychotherapy of parenthood'.

When parents bring their children to child mental health services they have not come seeking psychotherapy for themselves. However, frequently it can be recognised that there are issues which might quite legitimately have led to referral to an adults' department. The psychotherapy of parenthood is a psychoanalytic approach which takes specific account of the fact that a parent or parents have sought assistance with the care and upbringing of their child and that in addressing this we need to be prepared to engage with the significance of these issues. In doing so we can be of benefit to parents as well as to their children. Through the course of Mrs T's involvement with the department I questioned if she might benefit from the involvement of an adult department or a different approach. However, she felt that she continued to gain from her contact with a children's department in terms of her primary wish – to be a good mother.

Mrs T had always expected criticism. This continued in her relationship with her own parents, even in being a parent herself. Lisa's behaviour had served to confirm and compound this. However, finding Lisa more able to accept and benefit from what she could offer and having the experience of being recognised as offering something good to her child by her therapist, she was able to develop a more healthily discriminating view of herself.

Further exploration unearthed more information about the profound influences which had shaped Lisa and Mrs T's life together.

Clinical example 4.2(b)

Lisa's therapy had to finish, a decision due more to resource constraints than clinical indications, but Mrs T remained in contact. She became pregnant again and attended on a decreasing frequency during the pregnancy. This period of therapy helped lay to rest some of the unresolved issues relating to previous miscarriages and Lisa's pregnancy. She was able to establish herself confidently in breastfeeding her new baby and enjoy this new experience. One previously unrecognised part of the picture of her beginning with Lisa came to light.

There had been some health concerns for Lisa at the start but one of the mother's particular concerns had been unsubstantiated medically. She felt there was something about her appearance that suggested a genetic disorder. She accepted the results of investigations that showed nothing identifiable as a congenital condition but she was not totally convinced.

When her new baby was a few months old, in seeing her new child in the cot where Lisa had been, she suddenly remembered more of the time immediately after returning home with Lisa. She remembered the midwife and her GP being concerned that she was depressed. But now she realised how disturbed she had been. She recalled hearing Lisa speaking 'in the Devil's voice', denigrating her. She was too frightened to leave her bed for fear of her baby whom she believed was the Devil.

Mrs T had suffered an unrecognised puerperal psychosis.

The children of parents with mental health problems have a higher incidence of mental health problems than the general population of adults. Although puerperal psychosis is uncommon, postnatal depression is not. This emphasises the importance of training for staff working in maternal and child health in general adult psychiatry. They need to be familiar with how different forms of disturbance may manifest. It is also essential that this applies for those working in child mental health. Given the complexity of both adult mental health and its disorders and child mental health it is unrealistic to expect that everyone can accrue extended knowledge of diagnostics and therapeutics in both. However, the need for this knowledge to be available in thinking about children and parents provides a powerful argument for multidisciplinary teams in which different facets of this are readily accessible (Sutton and Hughes 2005: 186). Undoubtedly my training in adult psychiatry and psychotherapy was essential to the approach I took.

Patients' and professionals' best and worst interests

Psychoanalytic psychotherapy is an exploratory process through which thera-peutic gains can be made. It aims to be of benefit by enabling better access for the patient to her personal resources. This greater accessibility comes about through decreased internal conflict, an enhanced ability to manage internal conflict and greater freedom for development to proceed. In offering it we are proposing to the parent and the chid that it is a reasonable and worthwhile path to follow but we cannot provide them with a specific itinerary for the journey. We need to appreciate the place of any treatment in the life of the child and his family and to discuss this with them. Given the therapeutic requirement of time and regularity, how will it fit into their other commit-ments, for example school, work, other family members' needs? When difficulties arise, how will we judge whether they are inevitable periods of turbulence or developmental progress, the consequences of change, and are not indicators that a change of direction needs to be made?

Some people seek personal psychoanalysis simply out of an interest in exploring and finding out about themselves. More usually they have experi-enced problems and have found their way to psychoanalysis, or have been directed towards it, because of this. Some people become patients because they wish to be psychoanalysts or psychotherapists and it is a requirement for their training. The candidate's personal analysis provides a particular depth and quality of experience of conscious and unconscious processes. In conjunction with other academic components of their course and clinical supervision this equips them for independent practice. It should also be beneficial to candidates in terms of any personal problems they have. The over-arching aim is that they are better able to maintain the focus on their role in their patients' life. This should ensure that they are less likely to make errors or at least more likely to recognise errors when they make a mistake.

Any exploration is a step into the unknown. The quotation from David Livingstone at the beginning of the chapter captures his wish to recruit people for whom the act of exploration could be an end in itself. However, I presume he was also ensuring that he and his party were equipped properly in terms of the personal abilities of party members and the equipment available to them. An essential component of this would be that participants were able to make good use of their interest in exploration by resisting the impulse to explore simply by going forward when it was too dangerous or other essential participants or equipment were unavailable.

As clinicians we need to find out about the people who are our patients. Our interest in finding out is what brought us into the field of practice. Our value lies in putting this interest in the service of these people. This does not mean that we cannot enjoy the process of finding out about them, but we do need to ensure that our interest does not override or distort our ability to act in their best interests. *Clinical example 1.2* illustrates how my own interest led me in the wrong direction. I needed to correct that error. When I did, I found that there were contributory factors that were outside of my own internal processes which were of fundamental importance in understanding Mrs T and in facilitating a change in her experience. This ultimately benefited my patient, Lisa, through the changed care her mother was able to give her. I had to understand that my interest could be an impediment or diversion if I did not rein it in sufficiently.

Interest explored

Sigmund Freud is perhaps best known for his theory of human sexuality and his propositions about the manifestations of this in childhood ('infantile sexuality') and the routes through which ordinary and unusual development emerge through life (Freud S. 1905). In seeking to define 'sexual', he considered 'everything that is related to the distinction between the two sexes' (Freud S. 1916: 245) too broad. Two further components were needed. These involve bodily experiences which can bring pleasure or displeasure including genital sensations but not excluding other sources, for example skin, lips, mouth, anus. In addition to gender and the psycho-sensual, the psychodynamics of relationships must be included. Hence, psychosexual development involves the complex interplay of sensual experience, similarities or differences and gender.

History is littered with the consequences of attempts to live life and ascribe value on the basis of very primitive differentiations – skin colour, gender, sexual orientation. The latter half of the twentieth century was marked by challenges to many discriminatory practices and clinicians have frequently been part of those contributing to the challenge as well as needing to be challenged. Homosexuality used to be a diagnostic category. This was challenged and it is no longer included. But sex and gender continue to evoke complex responses.

'Intersex disorders' are an uncommon group of disorders. In some cases they may be immediately recognised at birth because of anatomical abnormalities. In others there may be gross physical trauma to the genitals or failure of secondary processes to occur (e.g. menstruation). Very rarely, there is unexpected development of characteristics associated with the alternative gender. There are six groups.[7] The following account is of the treatment and follow-up of the first young person I met with one of these conditions (additional discussion is included in Sutton 1998a).

Clinical example 4.3(a)

I first met Lesley when she was in her early teens. At birth there were no concerns about her health. However an abnormality of her genitals was recognised in her pre-school years. Her parents were not able to give me clear details about this, only that she had had an operation to alter the shape of her external genitalia. They remembered being told that Lesley might have some issues related to sexual development. They thought this meant she would grow up to be homosexual. They had not been able to seek further details or clarification and none had been spontaneously forthcoming. When she reached her teens, Lisa's voice had deepened, her facial features coarsened and her external genitalia had grown and had an unusual form. She was given a definitive diagnosis of Partial Androgen Insensitivity Syndrome (formerly known as Incomplete Testicular Feminization).

Lesley was referred for psychiatric assessment because of depressive symptoms, including suicidal ideation, and because she had described having confusion about her sexual feelings, experiencing erotic thoughts and feelings about both boys and girls.

In the initial diagnostic consultation, Lesley spontaneously talked about her medical and emotional difficulties, coming across as warm and engaging. She told me she could not have children so she thought it was particularly important to do well at school. As in most consultations with young adolescent girls, the ups and downs of peer relationships preoccupied her. She did have a group of friends but she felt lonely and isolated at times because of her condition. In parallel with her worries about her medical condition and what treatment she would need, her interests were similar to those of most other young teenage girls.

Looking at her, taking in her facial features, demeanour and clothes, I saw a young teenage boy: her voice was also that of a young teenage boy. I was simultaneously being presented with things which felt 'typical' of a teenage boy and of a teenage girl. At the point in the interview when I brought together the sights and sound of Lesley with the content of her interests and preoccupations – the former masculine, the latter feminine – I felt as though I had been physically hit across the side of the head – momentarily, it was completely disorientating.

I offered Lesley psychotherapy since she was already clearly vulnerable to episodes of depression and she was about to undergo a period of complex medical and surgical treatment whilst negotiating adolescence. A non-medical member of the child psychiatry team arranged to see her parents. Since no other psychiatrist was available and because of the complex medical condition I took responsibility for liaison with surgical and endocrinology colleagues. In the first year I could only see her once a week but I was able to increase this to twice a week in the second year. However after two years Lesley terminated treatment against my advice. During this time the major components of her surgery and hormonal treatment were initiated and/or completed.[8]

I left it open for her to contact me subsequently if she needed further help or to let me know how things were going. Her parents remained extremely thoughtful and helpful in their support of Lesley and with their encouragement she was able to make use of further contact through to early adulthood.

Clinical example 4.3(b)

After a few sessions Lesley told me 'I want to be a girl'. She had never stated this to anyone before. She explained that she had been told by her mother not to set her heart on being either a boy or a girl in case she could not be what she wanted. So she never told anyone.

The impact of the way in which other people saw her needed very careful thought. This was encapsulated in a particular incident. On a school trip she found herself with a mixture of familiar and unfamiliar people. One evening, a message was passed to her that a girl at the other end of the bar 'really fancied that boy'. When the girl was told Lesley was a girl, she was extremely embarrassed. Lesley described this to me without any note of embarrassment either at the time or in recounting the incident: indeed there was a note of triumph and glee.

Pleasure in another's discomfiture, *schadenfreude*, was a characteristic feature of some of her responses when issues relating to gender arose but not in other aspects of relationships at that time. Indeed she was concerned for the welfare of others. Where others might have felt intense embarrassment or even shame, she did not. In fact the other person in the interaction was left with these feelings. Defence mechanisms meant that feelings which would have otherwise been overwhelming for Lesley were split off and projected into another person. In addition to appreciating this defensive function, I needed to bear in mind that there could also be an aggressive side. She was capable of wishing to cause discomfort and of taking pleasure in it.[9]

As her physical treatment and her psychotherapy progressed, the psychological processes which were in operation changed. This was contributed to by a mixture of psychological maturation and psychotherapeutic gains and a response to the reality of the changes in her physical attributes. Her physical appearance had previously supported *schadenfreude* as a defensive process but now could not support it in the same way. Instead Lesley experienced her raw emotions and she entered a period of emotional turmoil and depression. Fortunately I was able to increase the intensity of her treatment at this stage.

Clinical example 4.3(c)

In sessions, Lesley was always inhibited about the actual physical nature of her body. However, she continually made references to her relationship with a boy a few years older than her. This boy knew about Lesley's condition. Their relationship was marked by arguments and making up and breaking up: it later transpired that there had been a physically intimate aspect from early on in her teens, but Lesley only tentatively hinted at this for a long time. However, continual references to him, allied with knowing her physical condition, left me pondering upon two questions. Should I be asking more directly and explicitly about the physical nature of her body and of her activity with this boy? Was she 'asking' me (indirectly or unconsciously) to do this or would she experience me asking her about this as intrusive – a violation of her privacy?

After further reflection I was fortunate in being able to discuss this with one of my old supervisors (Juliet Hopkins). She had not dealt with a directly comparable situation but her comments enabled me to decide to describe these issues to Lesley.

Clinical example 4.3(d)

I explained the issue to Lesley. She did not give a direct answer or response, nor had I expected this to be the outcome. It had needed to be made explicit as a reference point for the future.

A few sessions later, Lesley described an incident with a girl at her school. Lesley and this girl had an intense but ambivalent relationship. This girl had asked a question which superficially sounded quite innocent: indeed it appeared to have been asked in a child-like way in terms of its straightforwardness. Lesley had felt furious and her fury persisted as she reported it. I was puzzled by the discrepancy between the description of the incident and Lesley's response. To my surprise I then found the word 'scopophilia' going round and round in my mind.

Scopophilia was coined in the translation of Freud's 'Three Essays on the Theory of Sexuality': it literally means 'pleasure in looking'. Freud described a process of investigation of sexual matters, including the genitals, through looking; he viewed it as a source of both interest and excitement in early childhood, particularly the early Oedipal or Phallic-Narcissistic phase. In the ordinary course of development, the 'energy' involved in this becomes harnessed to promote learning about the world generally and in appreciating it rather than remaining fixated around the genitals and genital activities (a process called *sublimation*). This occurs through an admixture of internal processes and socialising influences in the child's environment. When present in adults in an unmodified way, i.e. 'voyeurism', the potential adverse emotional impact of shame and outrage in those who may be looked at covertly or surreptitiously are strong enough for it to be considered a criminal activity.

Bettelheim (1985: 90–1) criticised the translation of Freud's original German term into scopophilia as '[a] monstrosity'. His comments had stayed with me, and the word always grated on me when I came across it. This combination of grating insistence made me examine very closely what it might mean in this immediate situation.

What had at first felt like a technical issue about the extent to which one should make direct enquiries about their anatomy and sexual activity with adolescents rather than waiting for them to take the initiative now took on a different significance. I thought my conflict and uncertainty was in fact representative of Lesley's own conflict and confusion. She knew her anatomy was unusual: she had an interest in finding out more at the same time as having inhibitions about doing so. Some of these derived from the ordinary ways in which socialising influences influence the emergent processes of respect for bodily integrity of self and other. However, for Lesley, this area of life had been full of confusion for her and her parents, with much physical and emotional suffering alongside the acceptance and warmth in family relationships.

The defence mechanisms which had emerged involved a process of others being left feeling confused, embarrassed and humiliated in identifying her as male and then being told she was female. It was also what had been operating in my first meeting with her when I had felt physically struck on the side of the head in juxtaposing her visual appearance, the sound of her voice and the content of her conversation.

I was led to the following formulation of the psychodynamic issues involved:

> At a stage when the sexual researches of childhood are at their height a new baby had been born into the family. This baby was a different gender to Lesley's older sibling. The realisation of their differences to each other and of the similarities and differences she had to both was a traumatising experience. Impulses related to phase-appropriate sexual researches were repressed and there was a degree of failure of sublimation into exploration of the world in other ways: reliance on

splitting, denial and projection persisted. There was additional trauma from the surgery undergone during this stage of development and also by the failure of explanation or of opportunities to work through their impact. I suspect that unconscious influences on parents and professionals inhibited seeking full physical investigation and explanation. This further isolated Lesley from relationships which might have helped her comprehend and contend with her condition, further compounding reliance on primitive psychological mechanisms.

Subsequent work with other children and adolescents demonstrated that this was a common constellation in intersex disorders.

Clinical example 4.3(e)

Lesley had two particular memories associated with the operation to reduce the size of her penis/clitoris when she was five years old.

Lesley remembered telling the nurses it was her birthday. It was not. Nevertheless the nurses believed her, did not check her notes and made preparations for a party. When her mother arrived she saw the preparations and, having been informed that they were in honour of Lesley's birthday, she pointed out that it wasn't actually her birthday. Lesley reported this with impish delight.

The other memory was of having to wear what she referred to as a 'plaster-cast nappy' and of having a urinary catheter. She described going to the toilet and seeing what might have either been blood or a blood clot go down the toilet. This had clearly been a terrifying event and, I think, carried the sense of mutilation in her post-operative pain, fear and confusion.

Following her comprehensive anatomical and endocrinological assessment conducted while she was also in therapy, Lesley and her parents were given a full explanation of what the further treatment possibilities were and what they would involve. Lesley was eager for surgery which would fashion a vagina and reduce the size of her penis/clitoris. However, the actuality of the experience was extremely frightening and painful. When I visited her on the ward, she told me she felt even more desperate because her mother had not been able to stay with her on the ward.

In her psychotherapy sessions a few weeks later, her distress in hospital came across with added force and with an extra dimension that was difficult to articulate. This led me to say 'I think it feels like you've been raped'. Lesley agreed that the word 'rape' was the best she could think of for the experience. It seemed to me that the unresolved and unassimilated sensory and emotional trauma of those early years re-surfaced with all their original force in this new experience.

The next few months were very difficult for her. She became frustrated and angry with her parents and with me. She was not able to work at college. Her relationships became more emotionally self-destructive. Her attendance at psychotherapy became irregular and five months later she terminated treatment. This seemed to be partially an attempt to assert her autonomy but was also a wish to split off and leave behind her misery and turmoil, to deposit it in me.

It was agreed that she could contact me to arrange appointments if necessary. In fact, over the next two years there were a number of contacts usually arranged via a telephone call from her mother. This was a period of extreme turmoil.

Along with the difficulties described, Lesley also had many strengths. This resilience made it possible for her to maintain her development emotionally, educationally and socially without there always being serious disruption. It was also manifest in her imaginative solutions to certain situations and her mischievousness.

Clinical example 4.3(f)

At a consultation approximately one year after the end of psycho-therapy, Lesley was working in a job below her capability but her relationships had become more stable. She seemed to have a greater sense of her own core identity, although she remained confused by experiencing excitement in thoughts of potential sexual contact with both men and women.

Lesley told me of the way she had decided upon to explain her physical nature to the women with whom she worked. She told them that she had had cancer of the ovaries and had them removed, along with her womb. Not surprisingly this evoked considerable sympathy. I could see the element of fact around which this crystallised: the undescended testes which were removed because of the high risk of malignant change.

I smiled and said, 'That reminds me of something'.

Lesley smiled back and said, 'When I convinced the nurses it was my birthday when it wasn't'.

Lesley also reported a dream shortly before the previous conversation took place. In the dream she was with a close female friend. This was a friend whom Lesley found attractive in reality: she had no problem getting boyfriends but talked to Lesley about her anxieties and insecu-rities in heterosexual relationships as well as sharing her excitement about them. The manifest content of the dream was of Lesley's sexual attraction and excitement towards her. However, in seeing the way in

---

which Lesley was looking after herself better and presenting herself attractively in her looks and in her warm humorous manner, I felt the dream was also an expression of a healthy narcissism: I thought she was learning to love her own body.

Lesley's sexual identity as opposed to her gender identity[12] became more firmly established and she felt she was homosexual. She wished for further understanding of her condition, the treatment she had had and the likely implications of this for her life. It had previously been arranged that she could see her surgeon again if any questions arose and that I could accompany her if she felt that would help. Along with the more concrete anatomical and hormonal questions, Lesley was also interested in what expectations she should have of her sexual physiology and function, including the potential for orgasm. In the meeting she pursued this in an unabashed way, specifically seeking to have from the very senior male surgeon a description of what an orgasm would feel like. As the process evolved and her enquiries became more intimate, insistent and difficult for even such an experienced surgeon to answer, there was a further trace of that mischief which was the derivative of her schadenfreude.

In keeping with these maturational processes, Lesley was able to capitalise on her wish to explore, looking to the world in general rather than formal education. Her generosity of spirit was also evident in her wish to be able to contribute to the understanding of people with complex conditions such as her own.

Summary and conclusions

Respect for individuality implicitly demands that each new patient is appreciated as unknown territory. However, there is a range of ordinary-enough presentations of symptoms, signs and diseases that mean clinicians can generally expect to be in familiar terrain. Vigilance and surveillance need to combine in order to recognise where there is true novelty if learning is to occur and to ensure that the clinician can apply herself to the patient in front of her.

A clinician's interest in her subject is what makes her of use to her patients. But if that interest takes on a life of its own, then it can become an impediment in the service of her patients. At its most extreme, such interest produces exploitation of patients in clinical practice or research activities; the importance of guarding against this leads to strict guidelines in this respect, for example research ethics guidelines, good medical practice guidelines.

When new territory, interest, complexity and the impulse to explore come together, the opportunities for transference and countertransference pressures and complexity increase. It is at such times that the availability of other reference points for clinicians becomes even more important than usual. The clinical examples used in this chapter are unusual. But they arose in the course of the usual activities of my department. It was possible to respond to their unusualness because a pattern of interdisciplinary liaison had been nurtured in the ordinary clinical culture. The culture had evolved through appreciation that complexity may be present in even the most apparently simple situation. There are many times when this complexity does not have to become the currency of clinical interchanges: patients can be helped without 'delving into other things'. However, early recognition and response can be a very important tool in avoiding and preventing further illness, disease or complications in treatment.

Postscript

Translational medicine is the process of taking scientific and technological advances from the laboratory and workshop through to their applications for individuals and across populations. Recently I have had the opportunity to work with genetics counsellors. Their practice is at the cutting edge of developments in the scientific knowledge of the genetics of disease. They are also the human face of these developments which bring hope and fear to those people needing their services. They have to work with complex notions of probabilities and risk management: sometimes they can assign precise figures but other times they cannot. But whether people find 'safety in numbers' is a personal issue of tolerating uncertainty. As one patient described it to a counsellor, 'When it comes down to *me* it's binary: either I have or I haven't got it.'

The ramifications of knowledge about genetics for families can be extraordinarily complex in what is brought forward about historical and current relationships in families. The emotional significance for family members cannot be underestimated. As scientific advances continue, the need for practitioners who can understand their meaning or at least accept their complexity for individuals, parents and children will only increase. The study of these processes, what is new knowledge and what serves to reinforce the importance of the old, must form as integral a part of translational medicine as biochemistry, molecular biology, pharmacology, materials sciences and so on.

5

DIAGNOSTICS AND THERAPEUTICS: INTERWOVEN PROCESSES

Life is what happens while you are busy making other plans.[1]

The previous chapter demonstrated two sides of 'patient involvement': the active participation of patients in conjunction with the practitioner's ability to remain patiently involved. When longer-term involvement is needed, this establishes a therapeutic alliance through which the origins of the clinical picture are clarified, the specific nature of the constellation elucidated and the factors which are likely to influence the outcome formulated. It is a diagnostic *and* a therapeutic process.

Practitioners have to be open to receiving all the available data and information. Simultaneously this has to be processed to evaluate possible contributory factors and influences in the emergent clinical picture. Contemporaneously we still have to be in a position to act decisively when required. There are pivotal moments when we have to avoid the potentially anti-therapeutic effects of impulsive action whilst balancing this against the potential to become bogged down or seek unrealistic certainty (sometimes referred to as 'analysis paralysis').

The developmental dynamics of safety

Psychodynamic microtherapy

Clinical example 2.4 illustrated how a psychodynamic appreciation of mental state functioning enabled me to adjust my responses for Tony. My aim was to build a foundation for improved understanding and hence better treatment planning: within this I took care to reduce suffering if possible. It was an iterative process of responses and interventions as part of therapeutic case management. This process can be considered a 'microtherapy' which may temporarily counter adverse experiences emerging from the inner world. For Tony this could only momentarily replace being 'frightened for his life' with 'feeling utterly humiliated'. For Mrs J (*Clinical example 1.1*), I re-established our working relationship by making a transference interpretation. In doing so she re-made contact with the real possibility of being respected for her wish to do the right thing for her daughter. In both cases my aim was to modulate immediate functioning in order to help each of them make better use of their ego strengths. This microtherapy can be decisive in establishing a clinical 'momentum': its repeated occurrence is analogous to the impact of the regular experience of sensitively attuned care in ordinary development.

The psychodynamics of safety

Feeling safe does not necessarily relate to the external reality of a situation. It is an internal state, a complex interweaving of a number of factors: (a) the reality of current and past, (b) the experience and personal meaning of these events, (c) believing that the resources to respond to events are present in oneself or in reliable others, (d) expectations for the future.

A sense of danger induces 'fight or flight' responses with their observable behaviour and physiological concomitants. The scale of response depends on the person not the event. An apparently innocuous stimulus can produce responses which would usually be expected to be the consequence of 'objectively' threatening stimuli and vice versa.

Juxtaposing objectivity and subjectivity produces four scenarios:

- a *subjective sense of safety* in a context of *objective safety* can provide for continuing safety if accompanied by an ability to discriminate between safe and unsafe changes, i.e. vigilance.
- a sense of safety in the presence of *objective danger* which is a 'comfortable' position but it leaves the person in danger because of insufficient continuing surveillance.
- *subjective unsafety* in an objectively safe situation ensures vigilance and mobilises fight/flight processes.
- a *sense of unsafety* matched with *objective unsafety* maintains vigilance and fight/flight mechanisms are activated.

These different processes can be represented diagrammatically (see Figure 5).

The consequences of the three states of danger are different in their physical, psychological and relational impacts:

	FEELS SAFE	FEELS UNSAFE
IS SAFE	**SAFETY**	**DANGER (B)**
IS UNSAFE	**DANGER (A)**	**DANGER (C)**

Figure 5

Danger (A): a state of *hypo*vigilance or even complacency with the 'advantage' of the absence of adverse physical or psychological effects. However, risk increases because 'he doesn't know he doesn't know AND doesn't know he needs to know'. In the longer term, this also undermines the ability to learn which in turn maintains vulnerability.

Danger (B): a state in which there is the 'economy' of no uncertainty; there are 'no unknowns' so the challenge of discriminating between the quality of different stimuli is avoided. As in state *(A)* the possibility of learning from experience is lost. If the state is intense and chronic or frequently recurrent there can be adverse consequences for physical health through physiological effects. The interpersonal effects of responding to situations or other people as threats can also lead to vulnerability. Potentially useful relationships may be experienced as threatening. In turn, other people's functioning may be affected through projective processes leading to their behaviour towards the individual actually becoming a threat.

Danger (C): a state of vigilance/hypervigilance. In being reality-based, it has the advantage of enabling the individual to mobilise their resources in relation to the danger. However, if persistent, it may lead to adverse physical effects as in *(B)*.

Excessively intense acute, chronic or recurrent experiences of danger may lead to the re-emergence of primitive defence mechanisms which cause a shift to states *(A) or (B)*. This merely changes the form of danger rather than providing any realistic defence from danger (see Figure 6).

Paediatric practice involves many situations which are extremely frightening for parents and children. Simply being unwell can produce changes which induce a sense of unsafety: the source of potential reassurance or actual treatment can then become a threat. A good 'bedside manner' may not be sufficient to assuage anxieties. Providing information to parents and children in appropriate forms and at appropriate times is essential but may still

	FEELS SAFE	FEELS UNSAFE
IS SAFE	SAFE	No ability to perceive change and adapt. No learning from experience. Somatic effects may have 'cascade' effects.
IS UNSAFE	No ability to perceive change and adapt. No learning from experience.	Somatic effects of stress may have 'cascade' psychological effects shifting the person into one of the other danger states

Figure 6

not be sufficient. For some children and their parents, familiarisation with the treatment process and setting may allay some anxieties. In other cases approaches which reduce anxiety through desensitisation can be helpful. But time may not allow for such processes, or the factors involved may be far more complex because of individual, family or institutional dynamics.

The spoon that broke the giraffe's back

Clinical example 5.1(a)

Helen was six years old and had suffered from idiopathic juvenile arthritis for three years. It is a serious chronic disease process which can affect not only joints but also other body systems. Helen had joint pain and stiffness and her eyes had also been affected. Deterioration was putting her at risk of losing her sight without an operation. She required frequent blood tests, injections and medicines by mouth. Until recently she had been able to cope but this picture suddenly changed: she became extremely upset and fearful particularly when needles were involved.

Preparation for her operation became extremely problematic. Helen had been told why she needed the operation and she wanted it. However, when it came to the point of having to take pre-operative sedative medication, she became so terrified that she could not do it. Helen shouted and screamed 'No'. All attempts at persuasion failed. Despite her parents giving permission for the use of physical restraint, nursing staff were resistant to doing this. Her parents were left trying to persuade Helen but failing.

Helen was referred, willingly, for psychiatric involvement. She attended with her mother, Mrs Y, for an initial consultation which lasted about one and a half hours. As part of my usual introduction, I made it clear to Helen and her mother that if she was able to talk to me then I would listen but that she did not have to talk. For most of the time Helen kept very close to her mother, communicating mainly via her. Mrs Y explained the immediate crisis, the background and the wider family and developmental picture.

I learnt that when Helen's symptoms had started it had taken a number of weeks before the cause had been diagnosed. This had been a difficult time which added an extra layer of anxiety for her mother about trusting her ability to recognise the severity and seriousness of symptoms. It also decreased her confidence in some professionals. As the consultation progressed, she described how difficult she sometimes found it to know what Helen did or did not understand. At times Helen's understanding seemed very good but then at other times it was clear that it was not. She gave a specific example of Helen commenting that if she had to keep having blood taken, there would be none left: 'Then I'll be flat and they won't take any more.' Despite her fears of procedures like this, Helen was always very interested in the process and keen to watch what was happening.

Helen became less reserved as the consultation proceeded. She made some direct responses to me and even a few spontaneous comments. She, like her Mother, was full of a mixture of feelings – anger, frustration, fear, sadness. She came across as bright but confused. She understood that she needed the operation – indeed she was clear that she wanted it. After some time, Helen drew a picture (see Figure 7). This followed the mother telling me that father no longer lived with them. He had left three months before Helen's diagnosis was made when there were no concerns about her health.

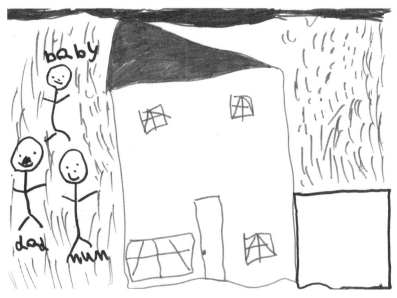

Figure 7

From the content of the conversation and the nature of the picture, I was left wondering if Helen felt she was the cause of her father leaving but I felt I needed to know her better before raising this as a possibility.

At the end of the consultation I talked with Helen and her mother about how complicated it was, knowing that the operation was essential but then finding it all too much at the actual time. I acknowledged that there were things to do with her fears that needed further understanding but that the urgent need for the operation meant that it might not be possible to help her with all these beforehand. I referred to the fear she had of having her blood taken, offering her the explanation that her body could readily replace the blood so she would not end up 'flat'. I pointed out an extra complication. She was simultaneously interested in and upset by procedures, for example having her blood taken. I talked about how it was difficult for both Helen and her mother to trust themselves, each other and other people but that being able to have the operation would involve 'safely feeling unsafe'. Helen's responses left me thinking I had made some sense to her: her mother felt that I made sense of their concerns and of the situation.

I arranged that we would meet again a few days later.

My approach was based in the expectation that Helen's symptoms were likely to be 'over-determined' – any one influence of the multitude identified could have been sufficient to cause problems.[2] Some of these stemmed from the 'simple' notion that a painful procedure could be expected to cause fear and resistance. Other factors related to Helen's ability to maintain sufficient trust in her parents and the staff as a result of real or imagined events associated with her treatment. Her parents' anxieties and doubts might mean they could not confidently approach the process which in turn might 'feed' Helen's own fears.

I anticipated that factors relating to her experience at the hands of others would come into play in the relationship with me and that this would take time to 'work through' – time which was not available because of disease progression. I needed to pay full respect to her fear **and** be clear that the operation needed to happen in a timely way. This would mean proceeding despite her panic and protest and being prepared to pick up the pieces afterwards.

Clinical example 5.1(b)

At the next consultation it was clear that the first meeting had been an important experience for Helen and her mother.

Mrs Y had been profoundly affected by Helen's drawing even though Helen had not said anything specific about it at the time or subsequently. Mother saw it as a direct communication by Helen of her feelings about her parents separating. Mother said that she thought Helen had been too young to have been affected in a major way by the breakdown of the marriage. However, the picture had spoken to her of how she had been seriously mistaken.

Helen spoke readily about her powerful and opposite feelings about her treatment and the eye operation. I reiterated my thoughts about the difficulty of having to have painful procedures and being interested in them as well. Watching her blood being taken gave her some sense of being in charge of things when so much was out of her control. I told her that I thought being sedated was difficult for her in part for the same reasons – not being able to feel in charge.

Helen told me some things that had been difficult previously when she had had operations. A particular event stuck in her mind. When she had been taken back to the recovery room her mother was not there. It transpired that the staff had suggested mother go for a cup of tea and she could be called when Helen was ready. We discussed how we could prevent this happening next time. I suggested I found out if there was any reason why parents could not be provided with refreshments in the recovery suite so that they were readily available. I then suggested that with her mother's help Helen drew up a list to take to the surgeon to explain some of the problems to see if anything could be done.

Winnicott (1971a: 9–10) described the potential therapeutic benefits of a consultative process even when there is no interpretation of preconscious or unconscious components of material. This consultation seemed to occur at an opportune point for matching Helen's ability to communicate and her mother's ability to appreciate this communication without Helen having to spell everything out. They were able to find each other without the previous sense of mismatch having had an utterly disastrous effect.

A few days later I joined their appointment with the ophthalmologist.

Clinical example 5.1(c)

Helen came equipped with her list. The surgeon read this carefully and thoughtfully with Helen. She explained what would be possible and took a photocopy so that it was available for all the staff. Helen used her mother's help to ensure that the surgeon understood things properly. The surgeon similarly communicated directly with Helen and used her mother to ensure clarity.

Having done this, the surgeon examined Helen. Observing this was very moving. Eye examination requires a particularly unusual form of patient–practitioner intimacy and an ability on the part of the practitioner to adapt carefully to the patient to ensure an accurate assessment. Helen clearly had trust in her surgeon.

Two weeks later, Helen and her mother came to the clinic again.

Clinical example 5.1(d)

Mrs Y had continued thinking carefully about the issues that had arisen. She had reflected on Helen's earlier life. She said Helen had been an 'unsettled baby' and wondered if that was significant in terms of her physical health, perhaps indicative of symptoms of the arthritis which was later diagnosed. She had thought more about the changes which had gone on in the family and how difficult that might have been for Helen.

Meanwhile Helen occupied herself with the toys. She enacted what she thought should happen after the operation, specifically that her mother should be waiting for her in the recovery room drinking a cup of tea.

She then used the bricks to make a tower, testing what made it more or less stable. She incorporated small animal figures into the tower, making the structure very precarious. Helen's absorption in this and her ways of ensuring that we took notice had her mother and I galvanised.

Helen put a giraffe on top and the tower still remained standing. She put a teaspoon on the giraffe's back and the whole tower tumbled.

Mother simply said, 'It's the spoon that broke the giraffe's back.'

Instantaneously mother and I both knew she was summing up the present crisis – the eye operation was the straw that broke the camel's back.

Mrs Y and I discussed this and explained to Helen what we meant. I explained further how I thought she was capitalising on the consultations to show us more about herself without it having to be that she could or should show us everything at once. I played with the idea that she was the teacher and we were her pupils: she was giving us lessons. I went on to describe how I was also a teacher and that I thought that the things we were doing would be very good for helping other doctors learn. I asked Helen and her mother for permission to use the material from our work together for teaching and writing.

Asking patients to participate in something which does not necessarily relate to their immediate care or have direct benefit to them is a source of considerable debate within educational and research ethics (Tan, Sutton and Dornan 2010: 9). My request took into account arguments such as the importance of offering an opportunity to contribute and the necessity for clinical scholarship in research and education. But my reason for asking them had its basis as much, if not more, in clinical considerations.

Helen and her mother were struggling with a sense of being overwhelmed physically and psychologically. They just did not feel they 'had it in them' to contend with what was happening. The approach I took had a number of layers to challenge this belief: (a) It engaged with the very real turbulence they still had in their internal worlds whilst presenting the reality that they were surviving it. (b) It implicitly demonstrated that despite the emotional turmoil and pain I saw no evidence suggesting they would not continue to survive. (c) By demonstrating the need for others to learn, it made explicit a lack of belief in omnipotence or omniscience in any of us. (d) In addition to accepting and valuing their individual experience, it implicitly communicated to them that they were not unique and isolated. (e) Furthermore, it offered an opportunity to exercise a generosity of spirit, an altruistic wish, without incurring loss.

My purpose was to counter the paranoid-schizoid mechanisms of polar opposites and unending circularity. There can be an alternative world of not-yet-knowing and of being able to learn and cope with more: a world in which vulnerability is not the end of the world. Relationships can exist without there being threats to one or other party. Mutual benefit and gain as potential outcomes replace the fear of losing oneself or the other, or of taking from or being deprived by the other.[3]

Clinical example 5.1(e)

Two weeks later Helen was admitted for her operation.

It was not long before I was asked to attend the ward because Helen could not take her oral pre-operative sedation. Both her parents were present and I spent a considerable time with the three of them. Helen was a mixture of frightened and furious, crying and shouting to be left alone, strenuously resistant to any attempts at persuasion or even the gentlest attempts at physical intervention. The nursing staff had effectively left it to the four of us to resolve the situation.

We physically restrained Helen which I found a peculiarly conflictual experience. I felt clear that physical force was required. I felt my participation was an essential and legitimate clinical activity. Alongside this I did feel partially constrained in the immediate situation given that I was operating in a clinical setting which, although not novel, was one in which I had not recently participated. I felt I needed to be conscious of the staff's expressed reasons for their resistance to physical intervention despite being puzzled by it.

Five weeks later Helen and Mrs Y came to see me in the clinic. The operation had been successful but she was going to need further operations. We talked about what had happened and there were no recriminations from Helen.

Helen's parents had discussed what had happened in hospital. An unanticipated benefit was that Mr and Mrs Y had been able to discuss their relationship and establish themselves as no-longer-partners-but-still-parents. In hospital, Mrs Y had found it impossible to think straight whilst contending with and containing her own and Helen's feelings. This led Mrs Y to further reflections on the evolution of the situation which had evoked feelings in her which were directly comparable to Helen's. Meanwhile Helen had drawn another picture (see Figure 8).

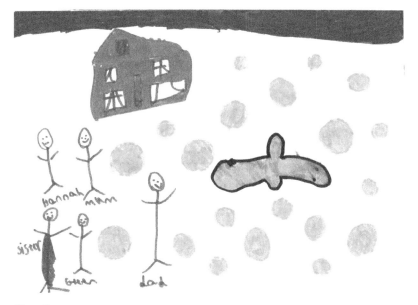

Figure 8

Six weeks later Helen was tolerating having blood taken without upset. Her joint problems were worse because she had had to stop some drugs because of adverse side effects. At the next consultation, Helen was much more settled.

I felt the original crisis could be understood not only in terms of the challenges of her condition and its treatment but also in terms of turbulence consequent upon developmental progression. I thought it was likely that where there had been reliance on primitive defence mechanisms more mature mechanisms were emerging. Helen could now know more than she had done about her own body and about her own relationships, particularly in relation to her parents. However, knowledge also brought challenges and potential conflicts, for example about truly recognising her own feelings about her parents' relationship. She was moving more firmly into the Oedipal phase.

This formulation was provisional and couched as an hypothesis since the more detailed data to support it would only have been available through a more rigorous psychoanalytic assessment or therapy. I also kept it to myself since the focus had to be on a *psychoanalytically informed therapeutic case management*, supporting her through the process of her medical and surgical treatment via the work with her parents and colleagues as well as my direct contribution. I was not in a position to carry out individual therapy nor was there anyone else available: explicit interpretive work would have required a structure which provided more containment and opportunity for working though of conflicts and anxieties as they became concentrated in the therapeutic relationship. More importantly, I did not know if Helen would need psychotherapy.

In preparing for the next operation I explained to Mrs Y that I thought overall developmental progression had been a significant contributor to the current clinical picture. I added that I thought two particular factors had helped Helen considerably: her experience of her parents coming together so well to manage her care coupled with Mrs Y's readiness and ability to reflect and learn more about *herself*.

In the next few consultations Helen continued to occupy herself with drawing and using toys whilst listening to and talking with her mother and me about preparations for the next operation. I thought the same predicament was likely to arise and that any attempts at persuasion and oral sedation would only prolong the agony of the whole process. I told them that I thought staff needed to avoid protracted attempts to persuade Helen to take medicine. Helen and her mother agreed and I wrote to the surgical team stating this. I arranged to see Helen again a few days before the operation and ensured I would be available on the day.

Clinical example 5.1(f)

At the pre-admission consultation, Helen told me no new problems had arisen and she was coping with blood tests. My discussions with Mrs Y focused on issues of trust and confidence – in staff, in Helen's body and in her own ability to function well and 'read' Helen well enough. She reflected on the times when she had not realised anything was wrong because Helen had not said anything was troubling her.

Helen reacted immediately to her saying this: 'What does it take to see if something is wrong? If we were in a car crash and I was thrown out and lying on the side of the road with blood pouring out of my head would I still have to **tell** you I wasn't all right?!'

Mrs Y did not react against Helen but accepted what she said. She appreciated the sincerity of her fury and frustration as well as the sophistication of her expressing herself so emphatically. She did not take it as a dismissal of her as a mother nor a total denigration or humiliation.

Through the course of a number of sessions, Helen had taken to doing drawings based around the characters in the cartoon film 'Madagascar'. This served a number of purposes. It was one of her ways of reversing roles with her mother. She would see what her mother could or could not do in terms of remembering and drawing characters. She was mischievous, telling her mother or me that we had got things wrong. Towards the end of the session the nature of her picture changed. Where everything had been bright and colourful, a grey hippo and grey clouds appeared (see Figure 9).

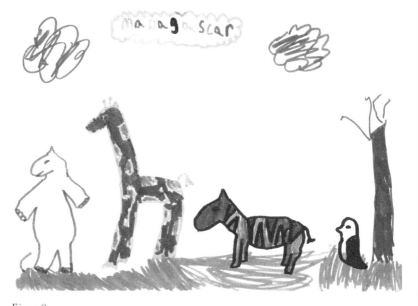

Figure 9

I told Helen that I had noticed the change in the picture – greyness and clouds – and that I thought it probably meant she was again feeling worried about her operation. She told me I was right.

This session was remarkable for the ways in which the routes for expression and communication about such a wide variety of thoughts and feelings in both Mrs Y and Helen were open and used. In turn, this was enhancing their own sense of competence and confidence in using their personal resources and the resources they needed to depend upon in other people. Playfulness and mischief were replacing defiant desperation as a means of discharging and resolving tensions, conflicts and emotions.

It was no surprise when the morning of the operation was again difficult. Helen did require physical restraint and she was given an injection in readiness for going to the operating theatre. I saw Helen and Mrs Y two weeks later.

Clinical example 5.1(g)

I went to the waiting room and saw immediately that Helen was in a lively and mischievous mood. She ran ahead of her mother and me despite the stiffness in her joints making walking upstairs arduous. She was clearly determined to get to the consulting room before us. I found myself thinking that I was going to need to be firmer with Helen. I had the thought that there was an element of her which was 'getting above itself' and 'needed to be put in its place'.

When her mother and I arrived at the door she had temporarily been able to lock us out. I unlocked the door and we found her sitting in the chair which her mother usually occupied. She looked at us with a challenging expression that said she was making a statement and that actions speak louder than words. I heard then that the operation had been successful and Helen would not need eye-drops any more. She then started drawing another 'Madagascar' picture.

I decided to address Helen's dash to the consulting room and displacement of her mother. I commented on some of the things she said about her drawing and linked these with our previous contact. I said that we were now in a very different position from at the start. Helen had learnt how to make herself heard. I suggested that there was also enough evidence for her to know that her mother had learnt to listen to her. I told Helen that I thought she needed to accept and appreciate that her mother could now be more the teacher and she could be more the pupil.

Later in the consultation, Mrs Y talked about how much she herself had been able to move on. Although we had not directly discussed how things were with her older daughter, Mrs Y had been able to help her by trying new responses to some problems which had arisen. She attributed her change of approach to things she was able to translate directly from the consultations.

The final consultation in a total of twelve was six weeks later, six months after the first contact. I was due to leave the hospital two months later. Helen and her mother had known this for a number of weeks. We had considered the possibility that referral to the local community team might be needed. However, the gains made had been maintained and her treatment regime had been stabilised without any incapacitating emotional or behavioural symptoms. There did not seem to be any need to continue child psychiatry input.

Helen presented me with literally the biggest 'Thank You' I had ever received (see Figure 10). Our final meeting happened by chance in the hospital foyer some months later. They were attending for a routine rheumatology appointment. Helen had had no new symptoms and her joints were less painful and stiff than they had been for some time.

Helen could be diagnosed as having Panic Disorder (ICD F41.0). This hindered her ability to function and she temporarily lost the ability to manage her behaviour, relationships and maintain her usual level of functioning. In relation to the latter, she can be considered to have temporarily lost 'capacity' in the legal sense (Department of Health 2008). In the multiaxial formulation, there would be due emphasis accorded to her disabling physical illness and complicated family situation.

The psychoanalytic model adds another dimension by assessing the nature of the symptomatic presentation in terms of its likelihood of being a temporary regression or indicative of a more fundamental disruption of development. Helen was able to 'catch up' on needs in her relationships through a process called *regression in the service of the ego* (Kris 1952) – 'retreat in order better to advance'. Responses which might at other times appear to foster a child's self-indulgence may provide the child with an opportunity to capitalise on other aspects of development to support the progress of other

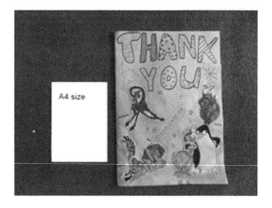

Figure 10

less mature parts or to process traumatic experiences. Regression of itself is not automatically a 'good thing' but Helen was able to benefit because of her ego strengths and resilience and the ability of 'the environment' (primarily, her mother) to match its response to her needs. Winnicott (1953: 115) acknowledged the difference between this approach and interpretive work but considered that 'The loss is simply that the child fails to gain insight, and this is by no means always a serious loss'.

I explored with some of the staff the resistance to using physical restraint. Despite professional guidance (Royal College of Nursing 2003) sanctioning the use of physical restraint if essential, the manifest problem was a fear that using physical restraint could result in accusations of unprofessional conduct. I made further enquiries and found that this issue was arising in other departments. The fact that a conflict was arising suggested there were institutional and organisational dynamics in operation. My sense was that the issues of trust so evident in Helen's individual case were matched by analogous problems within the hospital system and that the resonances contributed to the crisis.

Psychodynamic change as an indicator of organic impairment

So far the focus has been on the psychodynamics of states of arousal and anxiety and how understanding these promotes better responses to different states of mental functioning. A range of somatic factors also produces alterations in mental functioning. These can be reversible or irreversible, static or dynamic (see Chapter 2). The key indications of identifiable physical factors operating are: (a) variable mental state, including marked lability of mood or behaviour, (b) impairment of consciousness indicated by disorientation in time and place, And (c) impairment or loss of cognitive functioning. At the most ordinary level, simple tiredness can make children irritable, lose concentration and become over-active. Illness may lead to regressed behaviour: high temperatures may lead to hallucinations or, in susceptible children, to febrile convulsions. Intoxication alters mental functioning: biochemical changes and systemic illness may have comparable non-specific effects. Anna Freud (1989: 20) described these processes in psychoanalytic terms:

> it may be the ego organisation that regresses owing to psychological or organic causes. The ego may even be threatened by complete dissolution. Many or all of the vital ego functions may be affected, which then reassume modes characteristic of early childhood, before secondary-process thinking and impulse control were established.

The Developmental Profile is firmly based in a psychosomatic model of human development. The person we meet in the consulting room is a product of the possibilities of their genetic make-up and the influences of their intra-uterine and extra-uterine experiences – anatomical, physiological and psychological. There is accumulating evidence that influences in life can 'switch on' genes which would not otherwise have any apparent effects. Development is a process of the genes and the physical and psychological environment being involved in the *participative emergence of form*.[4]

The defence mechanisms available to balance the demands of both the internal world and the external world are inextricably interwoven with cognitive development. They emerge in a sequential way such that a *developmental line* can be identified and contribute to the formulation of the Developmental Profile (Freud A. 1980). In conjunction with this, Anna Freud also developed a system for 'cross-referencing' manifest symptomatology with the unconscious mental processes which she proposed were operative: her aim was to make it possible to distinguish between superficially similar problems in terms of the severity of disorder present in the child (Freud A. 1970).

The intertwining manifestations of psychological and somatic life mean that alteration in one sphere can indicate that attention needs to be re-focused on the other. The clinical case example that follows demonstrates the complexity of interactions which may need to be considered in the care of children with conditions that have effects on whole bodily functioning (Sutton 2002).

Clinical example 5.2(a)

Overview: Jenny was eight years old when referred for psychiatric assessment by her paediatrician. She had been born with a serious deficiency of her immune system, which was diagnosed in the first few months of life. For most of her life she had required once-monthly treatment with injections. Shortly before referral she had been put on a new injection which was administered once every three weeks.

I was asked to see her because she was eating poorly; her weight had not risen during the previous two years. Behaviour therapy had been unsuccessful. Simultaneously, she had developed an acute inflammatory condition of her eyes. At school she was having great difficulty leaving her mother and she was said to be underachieving academically. Following assessment, I recommended that Jenny have psychotherapy in conjunction with concurrent work with her parents and close liaison with her other treating doctors.

Jenny's eye problems became chronic. The differential diagnosis of her visual symptoms and signs became a major theme. Her general health was better for nearly a year but shortly after her ninth birthday there was deterioration. No specific diagnosis was immediately apparent but it was thought that she had probably developed a chronic underlying

---

condition such as tuberculosis. Contemporaneously, her behaviour changed: this included uncharacteristic rudeness to people. Further investigation required transfer to a specialist hospital. I liaised with the mental health team there, explaining my involvement and emphasising her emotional difficulties and acute mental state changes which had occurred (see below). After transfer she began eating well, her mood was described as improved and at times 'euphoric' and she was not being rude to people. She was found to have a chronic low-grade fungal infection of the cerebrospinal fluid. After treatment Jenny was well enough to return but within days she became acutely ill and was diagnosed with meningitis and septicaemia. In the course of this she suffered massive cerebral injury and, 16 months after the original psychiatric referral, Jenny died.

Jenny's case is unusual but the material presented below illustrates the difficulty of disentangling the meaning of symptoms and signs when there are multiple factors involved. A 'snap-shot' of someone's physical and mental state could have completely opposite significances which can only be clarified with the help of observation over time and finding out what does and does not change. Sometimes this can only be through continuing contact but a reliable historical account can provide the necessary information. For example, Jenny was indeed feeling happier when she was described as being 'elated': it was also less distressing to be with her in this state, particularly if you were not aware of the full picture. However, taken in conjunction with other mental state observations which will be described, the picture was further evidence of deterioration.

Clinical example 5.2(b)

During the first six weeks of her therapy, Jenny became less inhibited and appeared less tired and sad. I began to understand more through observing her demeanour and activity. She was able to tell me things but this was usually in response to my comments and enquiries rather than being spontaneous. Jenny's mother reported her as being livelier. For the first time in her memory, she had heard Jenny say 'I'm hungry'. Her weight was correspondingly increasing.

Over the next few months some things were easier but difficulties continued. Jenny's eye problems became worse and it became apparent this might be an adverse side effect of the treatment for her immune deficiency. The physicians had to balance the risk to her eyesight with the risk of infection. They decided that the treatments available to counteract any infections, should they occur, meant that it was reasonable to stop the infusions for a time.

Jenny also complained of muscle pains. It was possible that these had arisen as a side effect of the infusions but it was difficult to obtain a description from her which could help differentiate between other possible causes, including psychological causes. Part of my psychotherapeutic role was to assist clarification: it was a mechanism for translating verbal and non-verbal communication and decoding symptoms for other clinicians.

Some of her eye symptoms could not be explained by her medical condition. The observations were that in the ophthalmology clinic, when asked to leave her mother to sit down at the examination equipment, Jenny would suddenly complain about loss of vision, cry and cling to her mother. This variability in physical symptoms could not have occurred from the diagnosed condition. Unfortunately this was initially interpreted as her using her eye problems to 'seek attention'. I responded with a firm rebuttal since I felt this was a serious misunderstanding which could profoundly undermine Jenny's treatment. I contrasted the implication that she was being 'demanding' or 'attention seeking' with the reality that she was generally undemanding and under-assertive. I said that I thought her behaviour was the result of fear not wilfulness. She lost the use of her eyesight in a state of 'blind panic', more formally called 'conversion disorder'.[5] I pointed out that this needed to be understood as an indication that Jenny was again becoming overwhelmed just as she had been originally when not eating.

Winnicott (1953) emphasised the importance of taking a clinical perspective as opposed to a 'moral stance'. Implicit in the use of terms such as 'attention seeking' is a demand on a patient to stop what they are doing because it is 'wrong' rather than to consider what may be making it happen. This is not to condone socially undesirable behaviour that one may quite reasonably wish to cease. What it does take account of is the fact that the behaviour is emerging in consequence of turbulence in the child's mental life which needs to be understood. It demands of clinicians that they accept that this is something they do not understand but that good clinical practice demands further work by them (and perhaps other adults). It maintains their responsibility to seek better understanding and perhaps to behave differently.

Clinical example 5.2(c)

At her regular session a few weeks later, Jenny looked pleased to be there but she also looked tired. It transpired that, of her own accord, she had got up at 4 a.m. that morning in order to see her father who left early for work, and to get ready for school.

She referred again to problems seeing things properly but in a different way. I 'teased out' a description. She was 'seeing' images or pictures: she showed me what it was like by holding her hands right in front of her eyes. These pictures were present in front of what she could actually see in the usual way. She knew the difference between what she perceived of the outside world in the usual way and these images. Between us, we came up with the term 'mind pictures' to describe them and make it easier to talk about them.

The *content* of the 'mind pictures' was about her mother dying. Jenny worried that she might get cancer and die or might take pills to kill herself. (Subsequently I found out that her mother had threatened to kill herself by taking tablets a number of times.) The *form* they took was that they were recurrent and intrusive, resistant to attempts to stop them but clearly identified as emerging from the inner world and not from the outside. I therefore thought they were obsessional phenomena not hallucinations.

Following this, there was a series of missed appointments and unpredictable contact. I was then told of Jenny's admission to hospital so I arranged to have contact with her there. Her health continued to worsen and she went into decline. When I saw her she was at the point of referral to the specialist hospital.

Clinical example 5.2(d)

I went to the ward with my colleague who had been meeting Jenny's parents. When we arrived on the ward we found the adults in tears with Jenny 'flat out' in bed. Despite her being unresponsive, I sensed that she was aware of my presence although perhaps I just wanted to believe that she was. I sat down next to her bed with her nurse and stayed when her parents left with my colleague.

I had not seen Jenny for some time and felt very aware of this. Since Jenny was either unable to be in direct communication with me or did not want to be, I thought I would try a different approach making use of the presence of the nurse. I decided to explain what my involvement had been to the nurse, whom I had not met before, in Jenny's presence. If Jenny was able to take in what I was saying this would be a way of communicating with her about the work we had done together whilst ensuring good clinical liaison. I gave sufficient information to provide a good summary without going into any details which I felt needed to be held in confidence.

Jenny still did not show any response so I then joined my colleague with the family in another room. The family returned to Jenny while my colleague and I discussed the situation. We then re-joined them. Jenny was sitting up in bed, taking her medicine and smiling. She had told her mother that she wanted to tell me about images of 'good and bad pages' she had been having.

I spent some time alone with Jenny. These images sounded like further 'mind pictures' and I asked her to draw them. I thought they could be understood as a mechanism for managing emotional turmoil and I made an explicit link between the visual images and the difficulty of talking about upset.

Two days later I saw Jenny again urgently because she was to be transferred to a specialist hospital at very short notice.

Clinical Example 5.2(e)

Jenny was lying in bed, weak but cheerful and talkative. She was too weak to do any drawings but wanted to tell me more about the pages of her 'book' of mind pictures. They sounded like the pages of an ornately decorated prayer book. She talked with an intensity and involvement with the imagery that made it difficult for me to listen and concentrate. She told me she was worried that she might die. She thought it would be too much for her parents and that they would kill themselves. Jenny told me about dreams she had been having and was clear about what was happening in awake and asleep states.

Jenny went on to tell me about some other visual experiences which were totally different. The description was of many different coloured lights which she said were like a light show at a disco. They did not 'come between' her and her external perceptions; they were experienced as part of that external world, i.e. they were visual hallucinations. Taken in conjunction with the alterations in behaviour, variable conscious

> level and mood change, I thought that there must be an organic basis
> for these features. This could either be directly from central nervous
> system disease or the result of the systemic effects of infection or a
> metabolic disturbance elsewhere in the body.

Following Jenny's death I wrote to the paediatrician who had looked after her
at the specialist hospital. His view was that it was highly likely that Jenny
had had a low-grade central nervous system infection present throughout the
final year of her life.

Symptoms, defences and diagnosis

Using ICD–10 classification, Jenny can be described as moving sequentially
through different categories:

1 F43.21 Reaction to severe stress, and adjustment disorders: Prolonged
   depressive reaction
2 F44.6 Dissociative [conversion] disorders: Dissociative anaesthesia and
   sensory loss
3 F42.0 Obsessive-compulsive disorder: Predominantly obsessional thoughts
   or ruminations
4 F06.1 Other mental disorders due to brain damage and dysfunction and
   to physical disease: Organic catatonic disorder
5 F06.0 Other mental disorders due to brain damage and dysfunction and
   to physical disease: Organic hallucinosis
6 F06.3.30 Organic mood [affective] disorders: Organic manic disorder.

My reason for writing to the paediatrician at the specialist hospital was
because I wondered if stages 1–3 above could have been contributed to by
unrecognised organic disorder. This was not to deny the possibility of internal
developmental factors or external stressors as significant, but because I was
wondering whether the changes observed during this time might have alerted
me sooner to the possibility of organic change. If I had been better at appreciating, in its fullest psychosomatic context, the diagnostic significance of
the psychotherapy material in terms of the defence mechanisms required to
produce different symptomatology, might I have actually been a much better
therapist for Jenny? However, it is a difficult task[6] and, although I attempted
it retrospectively, I could not complete it. My pragmatic conclusion was that
in an analogous way to mental state variability, fluctuations in the therapeutic process and unexpected variability of symptomatology should lead to
consideration of organic causes. Such constellations are likely to be rare, but if

they may lead to earlier recognition and treatment, they may lead to a better outcome than we achieved for Jenny.

Wanting to be dead feelings

The preceding sections have involved situations in which the patient's safety has been compromised by identifiable physical illness. However, one of the most common areas of liaison work is the acute care of young pre-adolescents and adolescents who have taken an overdose of prescribed or non-prescribed drugs, knowing that this can cause harm and without an expectation that they have properties associated with 'recreational drugs'.

The immediate task is to ensure the young person's physical safety, taking proper account of any pharmacological effects of the drugs and any factors that suggest they are at continuing risk from their own actions. Most often the physical effects are minimal or readily treated. In the UK it is recommended that admission to a general paediatric or adolescent ward is automatic (Royal College of Psychiatrists 1998 and 2009). If sedative drugs were taken or if the young person is very tired, for example if admission and initial treatment took place through the night, direct contact with her for psychiatric interview may need to be delayed. However, information important to the assessment is still available through the observations of paediatric staff and through contact with parents or other carers.

An overdose indicates the need for a depth of assessment and after-care that goes beyond the crisis management of an acute hospital admission. However, it is recognised that building the foundations for such a therapeutic alliance is difficult (Litt, Cuskey and Rudd 1983; Taylor and Stansfeld 1984). Establishing an environment for engagement starts from the beginning of professional contacts. The contact could be with a person answering the emergency phone number, an ambulance driver, paramedic or a hospital receptionist. A culture of non-judgementalism, acceptance of the patient's predicament and recognition of a responsibility to act to ensure her safety has to be created. The mental health practitioner arrives on the scene when many other professional contacts have already been made and these may prove decisive in whether a fruitful intervention can be made. The psychiatric intervention starts with the care of the body.

My own experience of working in this field started as a newly qualified doctor responsible for treating pharmacological effects and continued as a trainee in general psychiatry. I found establishing any sense of a joint endeavour with the patient was difficult in the setting of acute care. Follow-up appointments were regularly not attended. The general psychiatric model of seeking to identify 'psychiatric illness' and people at 'high risk' of repetition of the act (and therefore more likely to belong to the group that ultimately commit suicide) did not seem fit for purpose. There was something wrong with the model, my practice or both: either that or the patients were simply people who could not be engaged. I was further challenged to reconsider my approach by a series of seminars based on the findings of the Brent Consultation Centre, London (Laufer and Laufer 1984). These insights into adolescent suicidality gave a radically different view of the nature of 'internal communication', 'interpersonal communication', 'suicidal intent' and 'impulsivity'.

What does it take for an overdose to occur?

The essential elements for an overdose to occur are the tablets, the drive to take them and the opportunity to take them. This is analogous to the idea of 'means, motive and opportunity' in the commission of a crime. The difference is that there is no criminal act and the victim and perpetrator of the act is the same person.

Suicidal intent

The law differentiates between *motive* and *intent*. Guilt or innocence is dependent upon what was in the person's mind at the time of the act (intent) not the reasons they may have had for doing it at other times (motive). Despite the ability, the means and the opportunity, the necessary component which could lead to the action may be absent or counterbalanced by an opposing element. Acts may be carried out because inhibitory forces cease to exist or become weaker despite the individual's 'best efforts'. Within the legal process disentangling motive and intent can be complex and cause confusion because of differences between lay and professional concepts of intentionality (Malle and Nelson 2003).

Clinical judgement is not a matter of proving innocence or guilt but clinicians do need to understand that motives may exist for doing something but that *acting with intent* requires something more. How we conceptualise motive and intent is an essential component of mental state assessment and is, by definition, required of an empathic practitioner. Consider the following two descriptions of the same clinical scenario.

Clinical example 5.3(a)

Mary, a 17-year-old girl, took an overdose of prescribed psychotropic medication impulsively after an argument with her sister. She stopped after taking only a few tablets and went to tell her sister exactly what she had done and told her to get help. On arrival at hospital she made clear her wish to be alive, although she admitted to having fleetingly wished to be dead. Preceding the overdose there had been a few weeks

---

during which she had felt very miserable after an abortion. Mary's parents had supported her through finding out she was pregnant and in the decision to have a termination but there had been increasing arguments between them. Her relationship with her boyfriend had also deteriorated. Mary had consulted her general practitioner who had reassured her that she would gradually feel better and prescribed the medication which she had taken as an overdose. Suicidal thoughts and feelings had not been enquired about at that time, but on assessment in hospital were acknowledged as having been present: however, there had not been any plans made to act upon these.

Clinical example 5.3(b)

Mary, a 17-year-old girl, took an overdose of prescribed psychotropic medication. The process of assessment proceeded by asking for a detailed description of where she was and what had happened immediately before, during and after the overdose. Working outwards from this, the background history was also obtained (as above). She had been struggling with how she was feeling but had not felt any urge to act on the suicidal thoughts and feelings she had been experiencing until the argument with her sister. Mary described how her sister had always been someone she could depend upon: the argument had felt like the last source of help to keep feelings of hopelessness and helplessness at bay. She had run upstairs and the tablets were there in front of her. She felt the only way to deal with how bad she was feeling was to be dead. She began taking the tablets, wanting to be dead. Within a few seconds she was suddenly terrified of what she was doing: she did not want to die. She then ensured that she was helped, feeling she could rely on her sister to make sure she was taken to hospital for treatment of any effects of the tablets.

Mary would not score highly on scales posited as measures of 'suicidal intent', for example she had not planned the act, her wish to be dead was transient and she ensured the act was brought to someone else's attention very rapidly. Yet at assessment (and in subsequent consultations) she talked about the period of time when she wanted to be dead and had acted decisively. Her actions had been with full suicidal intent. She acted equally decisively when the wish to be alive took charge and the over-riding power of the wish to be dead diminished. To have attempted to engage with her on any other basis would have been to display a lack of empathy by denying her experience of life.

My consultations with Mary were in context of having decided that I would introduce myself as 'a doctor who saw people who had tried to kill themselves' and proceeding by asking them to tell me in as much detail as possible what had happened. My aim was to try and gain as clear an account as possible but it also offered an opportunity for a form of 'debriefing'. As part of an overall change in approach, this led to very different conversations with adolescents about 'wanting to be dead feelings' and 'wanting to be alive feelings'. Only rarely have any adolescents said they had *not* wanted to kill themselves at the time of taking their overdose of tablets. In such cases, I still sought as detailed an account as possible and looked to examine the process with them.

Clinical example 5.4

Darren had not told anyone what he had done until some hours after his overdose. When I saw him on the ward he was quiet and apathetic. He was able to cooperate by giving an account but seemed rather disengaged. He told me that he hadn't particularly wanted to kill himself but when I enquired further he did say that he believed the tablets could kill him.

I took up the question of why he had not done something to make himself safe. It appeared to me that Darren had at least a part of himself that was prepared to accept death as an outcome: this made sense to Darren as well. For some time he had been finding his life difficult and intolerable. He could not see any solutions coming from his own or anyone else's efforts: he had experienced some suicidal thoughts and feelings. His apathy seemed to be a manifestation of hopelessness without him having experienced any 'pressure' towards acting on his suicidal thoughts and feelings until the immediate precipitants of the overdose.

The idea that 'suicidal intent' is either present or absent, weak or strong does not allow of the possibility that the wish to be alive and the wish to be dead can co-exist. Mary had very strong wishes towards living and towards dying. Darren did not have strong wishes either way. However, in both cases, 'wanting to be dead feelings' governed their actions long enough for the act to occur. When we assess why an overdose has occurred or the risk of repetition, we are trying to understand the *dynamic* between the 'wanting to be dead feelings' and the 'wanting to be alive feelings' and what internal factors come into play as a result. We are trying to judge which assumes dominance and has sufficient vitality for an action to occur or be suppressed. The period of time for which this constellation comes together does not negate the event or what the person experienced in carrying it out. Assisting that person to live with the reality of what they have done without disabling psychological consequences should be part of the clinical aspiration.

A cry for help?

To approach Susan on the basis that her action was a 'cry for help' would also have been a denial of the nature of the act. She had sought help beforehand and she did so again immediately afterwards but at the time, in her mind, there was nothing and no one to help. Susan had no conscious wish to communicate her distress. Contrast this with Justin whose mother is described in *Clinical example 1.1*.

Clinical example 5.5

Justin was 11 years old when he took an overdose. The family's situation had been very difficult for a long time and the relationship between Justin and his mother was extremely hostile. In the course of another furious argument, he said he wished he was dead.

His mother said 'Go on then. Do it'.

Justin went into the kitchen to the cupboard where he knew the tablets were. He returned to his mother and started taking them in front of her. His mother did nothing to stop him. Neither did she seek immediate medical attention for him although she did bring him to hospital some time later.

At assessment, Justin made it clear that he had hoped his mother would understand his desperation and hopelessness and do something to stop him.

Justin communicated his need and wish for help. Despite the difficulties between him and his mother he retained the hope that his mother would act to ensure his safety. His mother's actions demonstrated the depth of her ambivalence towards him. She was not simply neglectful; her action was hateful: luckily, something did tip the balance in favour of her taking action to make sure Justin was safe. Understanding Justin's predicament meant appreciating how desperate he was to keep alive the hope of having a mother who could and would do the right thing for him: he wanted to give her another chance.

An overdose is sometimes construed as a way of trying to 'get at' or manipulate another person. Justin's actions could be interpreted as an angry response to his mother, an attack on her. In therapy it might also come to light that there was an *unconscious* wish to hurt his mother or even a murderous rage towards her. However, to translate this into the act itself being an attack on the *real, external mother* would have been to deny the reality that forces in Justin acted to ensure that he did not physically attack his mother.

Young people who have experienced suicidal thoughts, feelings or impulses may in fact explain that they resisted acting on them because they did not want to cause upset to their family. Sometimes, having taken an overdose and observed the impact, they put it forward as something that they think will prevent future suicidal behaviour. In some instances it does occur that a significant person in their lives is present in young people's minds at the point of taking an overdose but these are uncommon: in these situations, the act occurs despite any thoughts or feelings about the potential impact upon that person.

Clinical example 5.6

John was 16 years old and being seen with his parents and siblings after being discharged from hospital.

His mother asked me 'Did he do it just to get at us?'

When I suggested that she ask him herself, she did.

John replied, 'No, I didn't do it to get at you or anyone else. There was no one in my mind when I did it.'

It can be difficult for people to conceive of the possibility that someone who is important to them and to whom they feel important may do something so profoundly affecting without holding them in mind. The constellation that consistently arises is that the overdose is taken in a desolate emotional landscape of helplessness, hopelessness and total alone-ness.

A 'psychotic' breakdown?

As described in Chapter 2, the use of the word 'psychotic' is not consistent across all schools of psychiatry and psychoanalysis. The Brent Consultation Centre group have described the suicidal act as a 'psychotic break' although it is virtually never accompanied by the hallucinations, delusions or thought disorder that would be characteristic of the state indicated by the word in the general psychiatry literature. The act *is* a breakdown of the usual ego function of self-preservation, but generic definitions of psychosis would stipulate breakdown of 'reality testing' which is not identical. In psychosis, experiences do not require external perceptual stimuli: imaginings are taken as factual without any need for external verification and will be held as fact against any possible refutation. What breaks down is the grasp of the repeated experience that 'end-of -the-world feelings' do pass: nothing lasts forever.

Sigmund Freud described love as a temporary state of madness, a state that can be all-consuming and in which the moment is forever (Jones 1953: 87). The perception of time passing is not the same as other perceptual experiences. It is not something with an identifiable sensory organ. It emerges in us rather than being a given at birth. However, it does come to be an essential organiser and point of orientation in our lives. It is not only disrupted by love: intense enjoyment can make time fly and displeasure can make it drag. Intense states of helplessness can also disrupt it. A threshold can be crossed which overcomes any ability to hold on to hope; the belief that the intolerable present can become a tolerable future is lost. The *persistence* of such a state is character-istic of severe depression which may be accompanied by persistent biological symptoms and signs including identifiable alterations in brain chemistry. Such depressive *illnesses* are very rare in childhood or adolescence.[7] But the occurrence of such a *state* is a further component of the attempted suicide.

What it takes for an overdose to occur...

For an overdose (or other attempted suicide) to take place what is needed is that: (a) the predicament is experienced as being insoluble, unending and intolerable, (b) the materials come to hand, (c) living feels like a fate worse than death, (d) the wish to be dead and ability to act on this are present for long enough and with sufficient strength to overwhelm any counterbalancing forces to stop this, (e) there is no reasonable expectation in the person's mind that an external agent can intervene to ensure safety.

The aphorism of 'means, motive and opportunity' can be translated into the clinically useful mnemonic of the *Four Ms:* motive, means, moment(s) of 'madness'.[8] (Sutton 1998b).

A psychodynamic approach to the crisis of attempted suicide

Creating an environment for engagement

The vocabulary used when people take overdoses demonstrates the different views held about the causes, meanings and significance of the act. Is it 'attempted suicide 'or is it 'parasuicide'? Is it 'a cry for help'? Is it 'serious' or is it 'dangerous'? The vocabulary used inevitably arises from explicit and implicit, conscious and unconscious beliefs about what is happening and these in turn influence the responses made. This affects clinical encounters and research activity, shaping the direction these take.

Consider the following two questions:

> 1 *Is the purpose of clinical or research activity to assess whether or not the person is at greater or lesser risk of joining the population of people who do 'complete' suicide?*

If the answer is 'Yes', a practitioner may feel a scale such as the Beck Suicidal Intent Scale is useful. (Beck, Schuyler and Herman 1974: 45–56). But closer examination shows there is an inconsistency between its content and its title. The expressed view of the patient about the act is not decisive in how a person is scored. Someone may state that they acted with the wish for death as an outcome but still not score as highly for suicidal intent as someone who says the opposite. So, who is correct, the patient or the practitioner?

2 Is the purpose of guidelines to ease the working of hospitals?

If it is, a screening instrument such as 'PATHOS' may be useful because it provides 'guidelines on the classification ... into varying degrees of concern [for] accident and emergency staff making the initial management decisions ... [and to] prevent potentially suicidal adolescents not reaching psychiatric help' (Kingsbury 1996: 609). This scale includes the Beck Inventory.

The dangers of using such scales have been recognised: 'Do not use risk assessment tools and scales to predict future suicide or repetition of self harm because the modest predictive value of those currently available makes them of limited usefulness in clinical practice' (Kendall et al. 2011: 1168). These tools have been developed because of concern for individuals, but they are in fact directed towards an appreciation of populations and health and illness care systems. Moving between an understanding of an individual and a population can produce errors and misunderstandings known as the 'epidemiological fallacy'.[9] They do not of themselves assist the establishment of a therapeutic alliance. I would argue further that they can act against it by institutionalising an approach which is not founded in recognition of the individuality of experience and is therefore counter-empathic.

Serious or dangerous?

The Royal College of Psychiatrists' recommendations (1998) are that children and adolescents who take overdoses should all be admitted to hospital regardless of the *dangerousness* of the pharmacological effects. This is derived from a view that any overdose is *serious* and indicates the need for careful assessment in a controlled situation. Physical assessment and nursing care demonstrate in a concrete way that the body has been fundamentally involved in what has happened. In that sense, the physical care is a psychotherapeutic intervention without words. In psychodynamic terms it is also an opportunity to provide asylum, a space in which some aspect of the acute stressors in relationships can be lifted at least temporarily. It is a demonstration of respect that something profound has taken place in the young person's relationship with their own sense of herself/himself. Just as we would consider an attack to have occurred if someone else had done something, we must consider the overdose the breakthrough of their own hostile and aggressive impulses turned upon the self. It is an attack she/he has *carried out* and *suffered* with potentially profound effects.

Not a cry for help

The longstanding view of the attempted suicide as a 'cry for help' needs reconsideration. The overdose is something that should be responded as an indication that something is seriously wrong. Simultaneously, it indicates that the situation was felt to be beyond any other help, including that arising from relationships. By the time the mental health professional meets the patient, the patient may be in a different state, but we cannot know until we have made progress with assessment whether or not we can be helpful. This is the case at the start of any assessment but there is even greater import in being conscious of this in this situation if we are to make contact with that part of the patient's experience from which they have been most at risk.

It can be difficult to tolerate being with someone's helplessness without immediate recourse to an activity. However, tolerating this without overt action may overcome barriers to engagement and be therapeutic. A course has to be steered away from over-identification with feelings of hopelessness and helplessness. Unconscious pressures to behave in omnipotent ways, for example prematurely deciding on and prioritising the problems to be solved, also have to be resisted. By placing oneself alongside the patient in retracing their steps, the patient can regain the 'capacity to be alone' as described by Winnicott (1958), i.e. alone but not isolated with no one to call upon inside themselves or in the outside world. Implicitly it counteracts regressive tendencies towards persecutory states of 'forever-ness' by demonstrating the timely-ness of what emerged and unfolded.

Mental state assessment

In seeking to obtain a history one cannot assume that it will be possible to obtain this in a clear and coherent form. Finding out the extent to which it is possible is part of the assessment. The observations and responses through this process constitute part of the mental state assessment. A hallucinated patient may not be able to tell you what they are seeing or hearing but their behaviour may strongly suggest that they are responding to things that only they perceive. Over time a relationship may develop in which he can tell you what he did not tell you previously because the voices told him not to or perhaps because he thought you were part of a dangerous conspiracy against him. Full mental state assessment is a process of serial present state assessments made in one or more consultations and perhaps in partnership with colleagues making other observations.

The dynamics of hope and hopelessness are central to the assessment of mental state. Hopelessness is a key indicator of continuing suicidality and risk of self harm. For a patient to engage with the process of providing a history, she must perceive at least a minimal purpose in doing so. Being approached to answer questions or give an account could feel pointless or may feel like just another demand. Not obtaining a history may be an indication of this rather than other possibilities, for example the patient does not wish to participate because she actively wishes to oppose the professional. In turn, opposition could indicate a number of other possibilities. Reluctance could be because the wish to be dead is persistent: the professional's involvement may simply be an impediment to getting on and completing the job. It could be that the professional's interest feels threatening because it evokes anxiety in considering what has happened and the patient can only respond by non-engagement, perhaps even manifest as apparent antagonism.

Being open to the possibility that manifest behaviour can emerge from multiple influences is critical. Appreciating that the clinicians' responses may be shaping this behaviour has to be included. If we can have reasonable confidence in our approach, then we can trust that the manifest behaviour is indicative of the mental state and integrate this with wider information to make a competent formulation. Evaluating whether the patient feels her personal resources or those of others can help is an indicator of hope and hopelessness: fluctuations indicate where the balance lies and where risk may be increased or decreased by concomitant factors. Taking time to see if any spontaneous expression of hope occurs makes allowance for the possibility of concomitant, different influences and can enhance the accuracy of mental state assessment.. Mary (*Clinical example 5.3*) spontaneously sought help and spontaneously talked about things that she thought would help without any denial of the motivation and intent behind her actions. Justin was clear that he had had suicidal thoughts and feelings but that he had retained some hope in his mother's abilities to love and care for him.

Where there is no spontaneous expression, direct questioning is indicated to examine whether the patient is in a state of passivity or of actively holding in mind the wish to act and waiting for the opportunity. Sometimes repeated consultations will be needed.

Clinical example 5.7

Fifteen-year-old Tracey was seen on the general admission ward after she had taken a dangerous number of analgesic tablets. She described a longstanding history of emotional abuse which had recently included physical abuse. She did not spontaneously talk of anything that she could see would change her life for the better. The story emerged slowly and Tracey appeared very tired after having been admitted during the night. I decided that it would be best to make this initial meeting

---

short and arranged to return later in the day. Tracey was much the same in our second meeting but she accepted the need to be in hospital so I arranged to see her the next morning. She was able to give me more information but this still relied on me seeking it rather than her offering anything spontaneously.

I explained that I would be making arrangements for social services to be involved. She did not object but did feel that it was a waste of time. Meanwhile she had begun talking to the nurses about herself and showing appreciation of their involvement with her. They ensured that I knew what was happening and kept Tracey informed about our conversations. When the social worker came to see her Tracey explained her situation. In her next meeting with me, she talked of still having thoughts that it was all pointless but now she started *fearing* that this might be the case rather than *believing* it. She felt that there might be an alternative to the fate worse than death of continuing to be in the situation she had been in at home or actually being dead.

Tracey's assessment and acute therapeutic care took time. At first it was impossible to know whether she was in a severe depressive illness state which would endure whatever was the reality of the care she received at home or despite her care in hospital. Further information from other sources was needed about the external realities. However, patient clinical observation and interaction clarified that the depressive processes could be addressed properly through continuing care outside the hospital setting.

Using information derived from the dynamic of consultations and the process of care still makes it possible to identify the classes of 'high or low risk', 'psychiatric illness or no psychiatric illness' or whether a patient is ready for discharge or perhaps needs specialist psychiatric admission. Such an approach requires time and a spirit of enquiry and engagement which is geared to the immediate patient. It is undermined by the pressures that can arise if there is an undue emphasis on a 'spirit of encoding' manifest in a search for categorisation or 'disposal'.

Seeking to ensure safety

Pre-adolescence and adolescence are stages when the developmental pull is towards seeking greater independence of activity. As adolescents progress this is usually matched by acceptance of this by those responsible for them. The extent of independent activity is negotiated implicitly and explicitly between adolescent and adults in a manner best described as *conditional autonomy* (Sutton 1997). Sometimes potentially dangerous actions happen because adolescents may only be able to experience a sense of their evolving identity through asserting themselves against someone or something. At other times, dependency wishes may emerge in the face of adversity or in seeking the advantages that come from not having to take responsibility.

Distinguishing between progressions and regressions can be complicated and sometimes they may be intermingled. Parents regularly negotiate these processes with their children and adolescents. They test when to allow or encourage more independent activity in order to help their offspring know more about their own abilities, learning when they have it in themselves to do something or when they need to look for those resources in other people. During illnesses, parents have to recognise when lowering their expectations is appropriate and then, in recovery, ensure that these responsibilities are taken back (Freud A. 1965: chapter 3).

An overdose demonstrates that a young person has been unable to ensure their own safety. It is their right to have their parents and professionals do all that is in their power to ensure their safety. Being prepared to act in this way sanctions adolescents in temporarily divesting themselves of responsibilities and can provide a better opportunity for further development. The enactment of this through attention to the physical care of the young person is an implicit expression and management of this process. It is a further part of the establishment of an environment for engagement. Allowing that there does not have to be immediate 'psychological work' on the part of the young person also serves this purpose. It is a further example of *regression in the service of the ego*. It is the antithesis of approaches which demand a rapid return to the highest levels of functioning: in many cases that level consisted of an over-extension of capabilities in an attempt to deal with the internal demands of development and the external demands being put upon them.

Assessment involves judging if the adolescent is able to engage in consideration of their needs for healthy dependence: accepting their own limitations is critical in making safe decisions. Similarly, being able to determine other people's strengths and weaknesses, including their trustworthiness, is essential. A youngster who is unable to engage in consideration of these may still be at risk.

Most often it is possible to consider with the youngster in conjunction with those in significant relationships with them the contingencies which need to be taken into account to have reasonable confidence in their ability to maintain a safe situation. It is at this point that problem-solving approaches will more accurately meet the adolescent's needs. A crucial form of question is 'What if...?' This can be applied to various aspects of their lives but there is a central importance on asking the question *'What if* you feel like killing yourself again?' Sometimes this possibility may simply be rejected, in which case it can be responded to by an honest challenge – neither she nor we as adults and clinicians can know that suicidal wishes will or will not recur. We can agree that we hope that they do not, but possibilities need to be considered if reasonable plans are to be put in place. Usually, possible activities or people with whom she can be in contact come to mind. The scope of this list is an indicator of the personal, family and social resources available to them. It is additionally an indication of their mental state in terms of the return of hope and realistic appraisal of these resources. If the professional services available are not included spontaneously by the youngster, then these can be stated and restated as necessary.

The focus of assessment is not only upon the individual young person. As with all child mental health assessments, adequate appraisal of the care being provided to them and the extent to which the parents or alternative carers have been able to engage with the components of the crisis and its management are decisive factors in the continuing care and the likelihood of progress. Occasionally external threats to safety or the failure of basic care mean that child protection procedures need to be invoked. Similarly, internal threats derived from the mental state processes may mean that powers under mental health legislation need to be invoked.

Continuity of care and after-care

Crisis management does not end when the young person leaves hospital. The decision for discharge is based on a reasonable judgement but it is its own test. Follow-up is an essential component (Kendall et al. 2011). Sometimes the possibility of re-admission needs to be called upon to preclude it being the result of another overdose: at other times knowledge of re-admission being available at a particular point of vulnerability, in conjunction with knowledge of the early availability of the clinician, may serve to obviate its need.

The first follow-up appointment needs to be as soon as possible after discharge if there is to be a confident expectation of attendance. The psychodynamic implications of the perception of time mean that delay will be more likely to lead to dissolution of the sense of the potential benefit of the therapeutic relationship. For complementary reasons, the appointment needs to be with the same therapist. This is important from the point of view of the patient being able to maintain the internal 'narrative' of their emergence from the crisis as a shared experience. The practitioner will also have a 'track record' in terms of the demonstration of their approach and their integrity in pursuing this to the limits of their role and ability. It is also enables more accurate mental state assessment and appraisal of progress.

Summary

The psychiatric and psychoanalytic perspectives are often contrasted by their different emphases on *form* and *content* respectively. At its extreme the psychiatric focus on the description of mental state phenomena may be viewed as being in direct opposition to understanding the possible meanings of the patient's experience or vice versa. In this chapter I have presented case material and an integrated framework which appreciates their complementary uses. This continues the theme of recognising whether our clinical role should be focused more on *modulation* rather than on *modification* or vice versa. The different emphases can equip us better to formulate what may be happening in any given clinical situation.

Embedding ourselves in a biopsychosocial approach provides us with a variety of points from which to orientate ourselves to our patients. A framework for practice derived from comprehensive models of physical and psychological development means we can better describe and understand the influences in and upon the patients in front of us. By integrating the psychiatric and the psychodynamic we can better orientate ourselves, locating our useful place in patients' lives. If we focus only on the wish to be 'therapeutic' we may not make use of an additional resource to our patients, i.e. the ability to contribute diagnostically.

6

MOTION AND MENTATION

It only takes a few ewes to make a path well trodden.[1]

Development emerges from the possibilities provided by the genes in the presence of a sustaining environment. Its pattern cannot be predicted precisely, but given a certain range of genetic possibilities and a good-enough environment, a range of emotions and behaviour emerges in a temporal sequence which makes possible the identification of developmental lines. Serial examination of these can highlight when the emergent trajectories are delayed, disordered or divergent.[2] The potential ranges of trajectory of the complex emergent systems[3] of human development are circumscribed by an individual's genetic constitution. Lesley's (*Clinical example 4.3*) genetic make-up led to partial androgen insensitivity. This meant that she could not be born with the anatomical attributes usually associated with her XY chromosomes. If different surgical interventions had been made earlier in her life, the clinical picture when I met her would have been different. The degree of response to androgens caused different patterns of growth in her bones so a masculinised appearance developed: earlier removal of testicular material would have precluded this but this position could not be regained. The clock could not simply be turned back. Analogous effects can be seen in psychological development. The presence or absence of possibilities may be decided by congenital or acquired factors. This may affect the absolute potential for something to develop or the time over which it will emerge.

More recently it has been discovered that gene-environment interactions can bring about the expression or inhibition of genes, for example cannabis use increases the likelihood of severe mental illness in the presence of a particular gene. Genetic influences mean that for some people there is a 'sensitive stage' in early adolescence when alcohol consumption could lead to long-term alcohol problems which would not occur if the consumption was delayed. Discoveries such as this mean that the previously polarised discourse of 'nature versus nurture' has to shift irrevocably to 'nurture and nature' (Sutton 2010).

Complexity Theory provides a framework for appreciating the components which are necessary and sufficient for complicated structures and systems to emerge, sustain themselves or change. Accepting ourselves as components, in relationships with other components, helps us locate ourselves, define our uses and appropriately accept responsibilities. We cannot always anticipate the magnitude of response which will result from external influences including clinical interventions. Apparently major events may not have the effect we think could occur: we then think of the person as having resilience. Minor events may have apparently disproportionate effects due to *sensitive dependence on initial conditions* (see Gleick 1987: 11-31). As illustrated in the descriptions of suicidal processes this means always being prepared to move between consideration of *absolute* and *relative* qualities and quantities of experience and their place in time.

The emergence of ever finer control over body movements, the ability to attend appropriately to stimuli from the internal and external world and pro-social bowel function are all examples of the synergy of neurological, neuromuscular and psychological development. They achieve major significance in children having a sense of themselves in the world, parents having confidence in their child's development and welfare and the demands placed on parents and other people by children.

In child psychiatric practice we work directly with children and adolescents and with those who provide for them. Concurrent work with carers, educators and other involved adults assists the provision of a facilitating environment which serves as an external matrix within which they may thrive. As with identifiable physical events, recognising psychological causes of difficulties does not equate to being able to undo their consequences. So, as with other approaches, practitioners applying psychoanalytic theory must not have unrealistic expectations of psychotherapy's ability to restore 'ordinary' developmental trajectories. But psychotherapy can assist in producing a better outcome where there are delayed, disrupted or deviant processes: it can contribute through its direct effects and the full use of the depth of understanding it produces to inform, and be informed by, other aspects of the care of children and adolescents.

Additional psychoanalytic concepts

Two additional psychoanalytic concepts need to be outlined before considering motion and mentation.

Developmental foreclosure

When there is a severe interruption in a particular developmental line, *developmental foreclosure* may occur. This is 'a premature but fixed pathological solution to relieve the pressure of anxiety' (Laufer and Laufer 1989: 172) which 'means that the developmental process has ended prematurely ... the ability to ward off any experiences that may disrupt the [status quo is impaired]. There is an absence of anxiety [which could] allow for any change of earlier solutions to conflict' (Laufer and Laufer 1984: 181). Developmental foreclosure differs from *fixation* where developmental potential is preserved. The latter will be manifest in a person's characteristic responses to stress, fatigue, illness and other challenges when they do not retain their 'best' levels of functioning. Foreclosure manifests without such challenge, producing persistent modes of emotional experience, behaviour and relating, more likely to be viewed as personality traits which will be apparent without stress or challenge. Primary effects can be detrimental through their direct effects on the person himself and on other people: indirect effects can produce internal turbulence and conflict as a result of the imbalances between different lines of development. The differing causes and manifestations form the basis for the distinction between character disorder and personality disorder (see e.g. Yorke, Wiseberg and Freeman 1989).

Cathexis

Cathexis describes how psychical energy – the 'fuel' for mental life – becomes drawn towards and 'invested in' particular experiences, sensations, objects or relationships. It makes survival possible by ensuring that the essential components for living are sought out and used. As development occurs different components are needed but the original investment may persist. If there is an adequate degree of *sublimation* (see below), persistence may not interfere with day-to-day life or development and may add pleasure to life. It can lead to creativity and mutual satisfaction in relationships. However, if the original focus of cathexis is not modified, it becomes an 'end in itself' and there is no adaptation to other needs or the demands of the outside world. This can lead to a psychical organisation, perhaps linked with bodily processes, which undermines overall development and life experience.

What makes children more active than adults wish them to be?

The ICD–10 categorises clinically significant degrees of greater activity than usual under 'F 90 Hyperkinetic Disorders',

> characterized by: early onset; a combination of overactive, poorly modulated behaviour with marked inattention and lack of persistent task involvement; and pervasiveness over situations and persistence over time of these behavioural characteristics... In recent years the use of the diagnostic term 'attention deficit disorder' for these syndromes has been promoted. It has not been used here because it implies a knowledge of psychological processes that is not yet available, and it suggests the inclusion of anxious, preoccupied, or 'dreamy' apathetic children whose problems are probably different. However, it is clear that, from the point of view of behaviour, problems of inattention constitute a central feature of these hyperkinetic syndromes.
>
> (World Health Organisation 2007: 206)

In the UK, the National Institute for Health and Clinical Excellence (NICE) Guidelines emphasise the importance of a comprehensive holistic approach to aetiology, assessment and intervention.

> The diagnosis of ADHD [attention deficit hyperactivity disorder] does not imply a medical or neurological cause. Equally, the presence of psychosocial adversity or risk factors should not exclude the diagnosis of ADHD. The aetiology of ADHD involves the interplay of multiple genetic and environmental factors. ADHD is viewed as a heterogeneous disorder with different sub-types resulting from different combinations of risk factors acting together.
>
> (NICE 2009a: 28)

ADHD is a clearly a *syndrome*, i.e. a constellation which arises as a result of a variety of contributory influences and has a variety of facets and the responses it evokes. It needs to be approached with the fullest possible appreciation of all developmental considerations and the range of behaviour that is considered culturally and socially acceptable.

Psychoanalytic considerations relating to activity levels and attention

Anna Freud (1974) described a developmental line of 'From diffuse excitation to signal anxiety'. Crucially, it is the line which describes where the developmental capacity to 'use' defence mechanisms in the classical psychoanalytic sense is present.

> ... in the early months of infantile life, pathways between psyche and soma remain open, so that psychic tension may be discharged somatically and vice versa. Somatic discharge pathways are not abandoned when mentalization is established. They remain available, with varying degrees of accessibility, in some children and adults mediating discharges that activate the psychosomatic component of such conditions as asthma and eczema. The early somatic pathways and the later psychic ones retain a variable interchangeability, so that the capacity for reversion along a developmental line can still permit the replacement of psychic panic by vegetative excitation.
>
> (cited in Yorke, Wiseberg and Freeman 1989: 6)

Anna Freud further describes how

> progress along the line [from *vegetative excitation*] leads to mentalised anxiety. Its first crude form is psychic panic of a primitive kind, which occurs when the child is plunged into complete helplessness and can be alleviated only by outside intervention. This is the stage

of *automatic anxiety*. Further steps in mentalisation and in ego development generally allow the child to restrict anxiety, although still pervasive, by crude defensive measures. Anxiety now arises as a fear of helplessness when the child is threatened by basic danger situations [*pervasive anxiety*] ... further steps in personality development allow the latency-stage child ... to use the danger signals to prevent the arousal of pervasive anxiety. This is the first sign that the way station of *signal anxiety* has at last been attained, however tenuously'.

(in Yorke, Wiseberg and Freeman 1989: 8–9)

The terms in italics indicate a developmental line:

vegetative excitation → **automatic anxiety** → **pervasive anxiety** → **signal anxiety.**

An infant's level of arousal varies in response to internal states, the impact of external stimuli and increasingly by an awareness of the world around them. At the earliest stage this is evident as total body movement, including the mouth, tongue and vocal cords producing cries. If we witness limbs flailing, face screwed up with accompanying wailing, we infer distress. Gradually the source of stimulation becomes better recognised as emanating from either the internal world or the external world. With neurological development comes more coordinated and recognisably directed physical activity until eventually language can be used to indicate a variety of states including hunger, pain, anger etc.

Where developmental progress is well established the constitutionally determined emergence of capabilities results in the 'raw' libidinal forces being harnessed, either directly for 'higher' purposes or indirectly by allowing an expression of the original object of cathexis in a modified form. This 'letting off steam' can give benefit without deficit and is called *sublimation*. The child's exploration of the world may involve greater or lesser degrees of total manifest activity. One child's exploration may be through extensive motor activity in physical space; another's through visual and auditory observation. One child 'takes in'; another 'acts in' or 'acts upon' the world.

Physical activity can give pleasure and promote physical health and development. However, for some children physical activity becomes an end in itself. It becomes cathected to a degree which distorts development. The desire and impulse may override other needs and wishes, producing internal and interpersonal conflict. In keeping with earlier descriptions of ego-functioning, assessment means examining and exploring the psychodynamic significance of physical activity levels.

The psychodynamics of safety (see Chapter 5) have implications for activity and attention. The aphorism 'fight or flight' captures the physical nature of responses. However, in the states described as 'Danger' in the grid (see Figure

5), the level of activity may not be commensurate with the reality of the risk. States of hypervigilance result in attention which may be excessively free-floating and non-discriminatory in conjunction with high levels of activity. Alternatively a hypervigilant state will produce the other side of this coin which maintains vulnerability through a lack of directed attentiveness and discrimination.

Persistent hypervigilance can lead to a state of 'shut down' in which attention from the outside world, temporarily, intermittently or chronically, results in the child showing a lack of engagement. It can be difficult to distinguish this from other forms of decreased attentiveness where an apparent lack of attention is in opposition or resistant to the demands of the social world.

Different developments

The following two clinical cases demonstrate the complexity of understanding and responding appropriately to the problems of high activity levels.

Clinical example 6.1

Alex was eight years old when he was admitted to the in-patient unit for further assessment and treatment. He had been diagnosed with ADHD, attachment disorder and moderate learning difficulties. Outpatient treatment had included the use of methylphenidate to the maximum permitted dose but this had not helped.

The multidisciplinary approach, founded on his nursing care, included once-weekly individual psychotherapy sessions. My role was to assist in a role which included some direct consultations with Alex in conjunction with his therapist, psychodynamic supervision of therapeutic work and consultation to the whole team to contribute a psychodynamic appreciation of the interactions and work with Alex and his parents.[4]

In the first staff meeting his nurses described how difficult it was to establish a behavioural program to manage Alex's life on the ward. Where they would ordinarily feel with other children that 'time out' was needed, it did not feel right because of the intensity of his distress. But they felt that a structure was required to deal with specific problems of him stealing and lying. Other observations were that he found choosing between things very difficult: getting up in the morning and changing between activities also caused problems. He would at times become incomprehensively angry. A particular incident became a reference point. When another boy came into the room Alex dropped a toy which broke: he blamed the other boy even though it had

---

been clear to staff present at the time that the other boy had not come near him. Alex was insistent that the boy had broken the toy.

My response was offered in developmental terms. I suggested that (a) Alex was living in a state of hypervigilance and high arousal and that primitive psychical mechanisms governed his experience of the world; (b) any change created a potential threat, so that moving from being an 'in-bed-person' to an 'out-of-bed' person, or from one activity to another, challenged him: similarly the other boy's entry into the room; (c) a crucial differentiation to make was that Alex was not lying when he said the other boy had broken the toy even though what he claimed was not true. He was not yet capable of lying because he did not have the ability to differentiate consistently between inside and outside, reality and fantasy. The boy's entry into the room had been another challenge to his functioning: he had lost the ability momentarily to hold on to the toy: this was the result of that boy appearing: hence that boy had broken the toy.

Alex kept his therapist on the move literally to contend with Alex's continual movement and climbing and metaphorically as he jumped from one topic to another. It was exhausting and left her feeling de-skilled. At times the approach of sessions filled her with dread. However, from this diffuse activity patterns began to emerge. He began using the materials she had provided for him to construct a game which featured consistently: 'Space Bandits'.

The central scenes took place on and around his 'Bandit Spaceship' made up of a mat and a foam cushion. He would venture out from here on journeys. He created a treasure chest from a box: different pieces of his treasure had magical powers. He had a 'necklace of invincibility' which he would wear and he selected items for his therapist to wear in the sessions. As 'The Commander' he constructed elaborate stories. In one, he told his therapist he used to be 'evil' because he had been to a place called 'Planet Evil' in the 'Devil Galaxy', but then he had found his spaceship and treasure and this had resulted in him becoming good. But then he suddenly said he had to return to Planet Evil: 'I have no choice'. He did not know whether he would be good or evil when he returned from the planet.

His therapist picks up the story: 'Alex spent a great deal of time acting and miming his journey to Planet Evil; this included a long exhausting space walk. He appeared to use every strength in his body to explore the planet and then get back to his spaceship. On returning to the ship Alex paused and became quiet. It appeared that this was the determining moment and he explained how he had returned 'good'. Alex stated that it was now my turn to go to the planet and now I had the potential to return good or evil. Alex spent a considerable amount of time enacting gathering something from the air; he then put out his hands in my direction as if transferring something on to me. Alex stated that he had given me all his powers to help with this dangerous journey.'

Through the subsequent sessions, he explored various scenarios in which safety and danger were possible and where he was a person who could be good or bad, making good or bad things happen. He was learning how to play. He dared to put his therapist in danger in these games – she would be ejected from the spaceship to be eaten by space monsters. As different scenes emerged, he changed the location of danger between different places and between different people, changing her into an evil person. But ultimately they were together in the face of threats and he made her into his rescuer, telling her, 'You're a life saver.'

His sessions continued demonstrating how he lived 'on the edge' feeling a threat of annihilation or of losing people and things upon whom he felt absolutely dependent. To need someone was to risk losing them so that 'having' somebody simultaneously brought fear of loss. In consequence, any relationship could suddenly switch from being supportive to being threatening. This also manifested itself outside the sessions and was discussed in the staff consultation meetings.

The complexity of his play and the sophisticated concepts he used belied his apparent learning disability. For example, unable to save the life of a character using cardiopulmonary resuscitation, he decided only his own DNA could save it: he enacted taking his own blood and injecting it. This character became his twin brother. His therapist described how he began to be able to reflect on things with her: 'Alex stated, "Words are powerful!" I agreed with this and Alex stated, "Are they... how?" Alex thought about this briefly and stated, "there are bad words that get you into trouble and good words that get you out of trouble." He stated that there were also swear words and that he swore on the unit "to help them understand how poo my life is".'

Soon after this, issues involving his nursing care became more focused around bodily functions such as eating and defecating. He obtained a toilet bag for himself – but his understanding was that this was to use as a toilet rather than to contain toiletries. This required some clarification for him and for staff.

With this better understanding it became possible to provide a better adapted environment for Alex including defining areas where there could be similar expectations of him as of other children. Gains in therapy and his ability to use nursing care were synergistic. His medication had gradually been reduced and was ultimately stopped with no adverse effects on his levels of activity, his attention or the gains made in therapy. It was decided that he would benefit from placement in a planned therapeutic environment. As the time to leave approached he was able to express his fears about the future and how he feared being overwhelmed by them. He was able to talk to his therapist about his upset at losing her – his 'very best friend' – and the unit. Rather than loss meaning total devastation and annihilation he could appreciate ''Tis better to have loved and lost than never to have loved at all' (Tennyson).

These excerpts illustrate developmental progress along a line 'from diffuse excitation to signal anxiety'. Alex's progress could be identified along other lines and using other perspectives, for example the move on from primary reliance on splitting and projection, his ability to learn in an educational environment and his ability to cope in groups. His ability to manage his own internal states was far most robustly established although he was still reliant on the sensitive attunement of adults. In the following year his progress was maintained in his special school without medication. It was still likely that he would need extra care at points of predictable crisis such as school change or in response to the more ordinary challenges of development, for example puberty.

Clinical example 6.2

Tim was first referred when he was five years old. His major problems were aggression and outbursts of extreme uncontrollable behaviour: these occurred at home and at school. The problems were attributed principally to parenting problems in context of his mother having a chronic illness with a fluctuating course. His parents requested a second opinion because they did not agree with the formulation and did not feel the interventions that were recommended were helpful. He had had psychometric testing which showed an uneven borderline intellectual profile.

The second assessment placed greater emphasis on internal developmental and dynamic processes. Difficulties in the developmental line for anxiety were felt to be significant contributors. The assessing team also realised that they would need to understand better whether parental responses which on the surface might appear to be unhelpful or even compounding of his problems might actually be sensitive adaptations which were beneficial. The complex interactions within his uneven intellectual profile meant that he found the ordinary expectations of the classroom and unstructured school time difficult and that he presented behavioural management problems. Individual psychotherapy for Tim and contemporaneous parental therapy were arranged: procedures to ensure his special educational needs were fully assessed were initiated.

Initially Tim thrived on an approach which sought to engage him in playful activity in the face of what seemed to be anxiety-driven behaviour. Although he had been able to separate from his mother, he hid behind curtains peeping out intermittently. I told him I thought he was showing me how he was not sure he was safe in the room with me. He responded warmly to this and then repeatedly enacted a scenario which involved crawling out from underneath a chair which was covered with a blanket. The link with being inside or outside and the form it took led me to introduce the idea that I thought it related to his feelings about being inside or outside his mother. Tim again responded positively and warmly to this.

A pattern developed of Tim climbing on the window sill, closing and opening the curtains as a 'Now you see me, now you don't' game which I picked up as a game of Peepo. Over time he elaborated this into opening and closing the curtains very quickly whilst insisting that I said whether I could see him or not. He did it quickly enough to ensure that I would always get it wrong. This was readily interpretable as him putting me in the position which he had experienced so frequently. Intermingled with these activities were other games, particularly football. He was skilful and well coordinated.

As Tim moved into latency phase he became less engaged and then overtly in opposition to his therapy, denigrating it and me. Some aspects of this could be attributed to phase-appropriate mechanisms related to latency but after two years of once-weekly therapy it became unsustainable.

The work with his mother and liaison with school and the education service continued. The principal task in the school liaison was to try and change their view of his challenging behaviour as wilful (and therefore something which he should accept responsibility for changing) to an appreciation of his inability to rise to the demands of their expectations. There was resistance to believing Tim needed an alternative environment for learning. This 'moral attitude' (Winnicott 1953: 104) was in context of a political and educational view that 'social inclusion' was tantamount to a panacea and that to recommend alternative education was to risk the dire consequences of 'social exclusion'.

Tim was eventually placed in a special school which was philosophically and practically able to offer him a much better environment. He made significant general progress but secondary school age arrived and a change was inevitable. The special school of choice was not possible because of financial constraints but he was placed in a special educational unit which allowed him to engage in more physical activity than would be possible in the ordinary school environment. However, adolescence brought with it increasing aggressive and oppositional behaviour.

Tim's mother was aware of my concerns about the frequency with which children were being diagnosed as having ADHD, specifically where this seemed to bring with it the assumption of drug treatment. She knew I was not ideologically opposed to medication and I had raised it as a possibility but for a long time she did not wish to pursue this line. However, as the situation became more difficult she discussed it with Tim and they decided that he should try it.

Tim liked being on methylphenidate. He could not easily describe the difference he found except that he felt a bit calmer. His mother accepted this but from her point of view she did not register any major differences nor were there significant changes in reports from school. In clinic Tim was able to engage to some degree but this was interwoven with elements of opposition and defiance. He was reluctant to talk and mischievous, for example in response to something I said, he stroked his hand over his head apparently innocently but with two fingers forming a 'V' sign.

Tim remained on methylphenidate.

These two cases illustrate the importance of being open to considering the variety of influences which can apply. Just as the Biomedical Model is deficient if it does not expand to integrate psychosocial influences, so too is a Biopsychosocial Model if it does not pay full respect to the biological.

Further developmental considerations

Drug treatment is increasingly being used in the UK, matching the extent of its use in the USA. The greatest dilemma is the possible implication for maturational processes.

There are children in whom there is a specific 'gap' where a pharmacological intervention allows for compensation. The drug may be a replacement therapy comparable to the role of insulin in diabetes. Drug treatment may prevent primary adverse affects and further benefit the child through avoidance of the secondary effects upon relationships and education. However, the evidence is not yet present to refute the possibility that children's development can be adversely affected by reducing activity and attentional processes pharmacologically when they do have such a deficit.

By returning to Winnicott's (1965) book title *The maturational processes and the facilitating environment*, and allowing a temporary indulgence in dualism, the argument can be explored further. Administering a drug is clearly an action from the external environment. It has significance in terms of the child's intimate and wider relationships. The physiological environment is clearly an *internal* environment, part of the overall system that is the person who is maturing. The person's psychical experience of these somatic effects has to be incorporated into the effects on the evolution of the sense of self, particularly in terms of the sense of agency. In one sense, the internal physiological environment is part of a facilitating or inhibiting environment.

When considering an individual's ability to manage levels of activity and direct their attention, the implications for attributions of wilfulness or lack of it are manifold and profound. To what extent might the sense of autonomy (of will and action) evolve in a different way because of the interpersonal and physiological processes involved? Might the use of medication produce an iatrogenic delay (or *further* delay if there is inherent slowness of maturation)? Even more profoundly, might it produce developmental foreclosure? This carries with it the possibility of potential cascade effects. Just as in the argument in favour of the use of medication, a clinically balanced approach must allow for any potentially adverse effects.

A further counterbalancing factor for consideration was pointed out to me by Dr Ruth Marshall. For some children who may ultimately be judged likely to benefit from medication, delay may mean that the potential for thera-peutic engagement may be impaired. If the emergent constellation includes oppositionality as a significant component there may be resistance to a trial of medication. Such a pattern could well be contributed to by secondary effects of hyperactivity or attention problems.

That guidelines advise against the use of medication in pre-school children can be considered a pragmatic compromise. It acknowledges not only the diagnostic and treatment dilemmas but also produces a situation which delays an intervention with a theoretical risk of causing a specific develop-mental delay or foreclosure. But five years old is still a tender age.

What builds is a picture of the complexity and the array of factors which child health practitioners (mental health and physical health) must consider when deciding whether a signature on a prescription is the most reasonable action. Given the multifactorial nature of the problem, undue reliance on simply titrating activity levels against medication dosage may not be reasonable. Making clinical judgements about the continuing care of children with activity and attentional difficulties requires care which is based in a comprehensive framework of biopsychosocial care. This leaves me circum-spect about the recommendation that the training of paediatricians (albeit *special* training) is equivalent to child psychiatric training in this respect as advised by the National Institute for Health & Clinical Excellence (2009a).

Although the countertransference impact of these problems has not been considered in detail, it is implicit in the emphasis I have placed on adults considering why they wish the child's activity levels to be lower or the child's attention to be focused in a particular way. Wanting to decrease disruptive activity or to increase activities which are considered desirable may stem from conscious processes. It may be a simple difference between adult and child about what is desirable or a realistic demand given the circumstances. It may also stem from unconscious processes in the child. Their need for adult involvement may be a manifestation of projective processes and their need may be for adults to contain their own discomforting experience through tolerance rather than seeking to restrict or divert the child's activity. Any 'attention seeking' aspect of their behaviour may be undesirable in ordinary terms but inevitable or essential in the child's world (Winnicott 1956b).

Until recently the debate about ADHD had been confined to child and adolescent psychiatry. This has now extended to adult psychiatry as the cohort of young people on medication has reached adulthood. In conjunction with this are those adults who could have been diagnosed in childhood and who have problems which could be manifestations of primary or secondary effects of ADHD. Further exploration of this is beyond the scope of this book.

Behaviour therapy: who is the patient?

Guidelines recommend including behaviour therapy in treatment. Its exponents will base the explanation of its value in principles of learning theory but it is interesting to examine it from a more Winnicottian perspective.

In common with psychodynamic approaches, a behavioural intervention should be based on sound psychological/psychiatric assessment of a child's state using observational, historical and developmental detail. A plan is then drawn up to match the child's abilities with the expectations other people have of him. Targets are set to be within the proximal zone of reasonable further expectation (to adapt Vygotsky's (1978) concept of *proximal zone of developmen*). Change is produced through the child being rewarded for performing on target consistently.

One can see this as paying full respect to a child's abilities, rewarding him for consolidated maturational achievements. In fact he is being rewarded by the provision of a facilitating environment, i.e. one that is truly geared to what is reasonable to expect of him. Behavioural modification is achieved by adults first attempting to achieve a comprehensive understanding of the child and then modifying their behaviour accordingly. For some reason there seems to be a need to perpetuate a fantasy that this represents a specific clinical treatment of children rather than treating children appropriately by altering adult behaviour to be better reasoned and more reasonable!

The power and possibilities of poo

For a child, mastery of body movements brings forth the possibility of a phase shift in experience. There may be simple pleasure in the achievement of mastery. As the ability to coordinate movements develops, the groups of muscles which might previously only have operated in opposition to each other can now act synergistically. From being someone whose thumb waves around in front of her face, the baby becomes someone who can insert a thumb into her mouth and gain comfort and pleasure from sucking it. Such an apparently simple manoeuvre but an achievement of major import in terms of the experience of self, sensorally and sensually, and the extent of absolute dependence on a carer. It is empowering literally and metaphorically.

The baby's bodily processes and reliance on others to ensure food, warmth and the removal of potentially harmful products are the foundations of parenting. Bodily sensations, the emergence of mastery of movements and processes, and relationships are intertwined from birth. The baby cannot simply tell us when she becomes aware of a need. Nor can she tell us about the discrepancy between her realisation of wish or need and the appreciation of who can do something about it. She relies on sensitively attuned carers, adapting to her needs, wishes and abilities, negotiating the vicissitudes of these experiences and guiding her as to what she has it in herself to do or not do. Out of these processes emerges a person who can know better what she has it in herself to do or not do – for better or for worse.

Faeces and defecation have particular significance in terms of mastery and relationships. Of necessity, the baby's bottom and its products are a principal focus of attention for parents. The child experiences her parents' physical care of her and can observe them in their degree of visual focus on her different parts. She feels what they do without seeing where they are doing it. She can see their facial expressions and hear their vocalisations. It becomes a particular meeting place.

In association with this she experiences her gut in its contractions, the sphincter in its relaxation and the process of fecal matter passing, usually to come into contact with another part of her body. Later, interest in what is happening 'down below' can be observed as she explores with her fingers, giving an additional cleaning-up job to the nappy-changer. She may want to look at what is on her fingers – or even taste it!

As development makes it possible to delay defecation and deposit the faeces somewhere specific other than in the nappy, their potential significance in relationships changes. It can happen at a convenient time and in a convenient place – a gift from the child to her parents. Faeces can be withheld, perhaps simply to see what happens or maybe in awareness of it causing inconvenience or displeasure. In conjunction with the child's imaginings carried over from earlier times, the possibility of sphincter control can prove to be a fertile field for mental life, of understanding inside, outside or in-between and in the exploration of power in relationships.

The attributions children make to their faeces can become manifest as they play with ideas,[5] make jokes or become anxious about what might be lurking in the toilet bowl – perhaps a crocodile? In psychotherapy sessions, children may suddenly leave the room, desperate for the toilet even though they went just before the session started. As the therapeutic work proceeds, it becomes apparent that defecation (or urination) was a physicalisation of the mental experience, an expulsion of anxiety.

Problems with poo

My work with problems of encopresis involved working with community and hospital paediatric services and a highly specialised surgical service for children with chronic severe bowel and defecation problems. Although a small proportion of these children had previously had identifiable causes for dysfunction the majority did not.

From both direct work with mothers and babies and from the histories of older children it was striking how often a diagnosis of constipation was made in young babies without rigorous consideration of the different possible causes for distress associated with defecation. This is despite diagnostic guidelines existing over many years and more recently formulated in the UK by NICE (National Collaborating Centre for Women's and Children's Health 2010). This guidance includes the statement 'often accompanied by straining and pain'. In babies we can only infer pain: we cannot really know the intention behind certain things they do in order to infer intent when they appear to be 'straining at stool'. In eliciting detailed descriptions of events from mothers, I would hear of repeated episodes of crying, sometimes prolonged, which would cease when the baby defecated. The faeces were not necessarily unusual, but the sequence

crying → defecation → cessation of crying

regularly appeared to trigger the diagnosis and lead to advice or specific interventions based on this.

Observing babies in states of vegetative excitation, one sees that they sometimes defecate and then stop crying. At other times they are fed and stop crying. At still other times, it is not clear what happens, but they do stop crying quickly or eventually. Sometimes mother returns or some other person takes over their care and crying stops. In all of these states there is crying and thrashing around, perhaps episodes of catching their breath and their abdomens becoming tense and appearing distended. The manifest behaviour feels unmistakeably expressive of intense distress without being specific in its likely cause. In some instances the faeces may be hard and it is reasonable to interpret this as the cause of pain. However, another reasonable explanation is that any process of intense stimulation will cause distress even in the absence of a stimulus thought to be sufficient to cause 'physical' pain. Contractions of the gut and relaxation of the anal sphincter might induce a change of experience sufficient to disrupt and distress a baby. The passing of a stool and cessation of stimulation might lead to a return of equilibrium, perhaps even equanimity, and crying stops.

It is not unreasonable to propose that at the earliest periods of life a child experiences pain or distress associated with a physical sensation as something that 'gets into her' rather than the result of something getting out of her. The primary relevance of the anus to survival is as an *exit* point but the localised anatomical area is the point identifiable as where pain *'gets in'*. How the baby processes all this and the attributions made in their imaginings will be affected by the extent to which they are helped by the holding/containment they experience. Recognising which is which can only come later and represents one aspect of the move from paranoid schizoid states of functioning to the *depressive position* as proposed in Kleinian theory (see Laplanche and Pontalis 1988: 114–16) and *concern* by Winnicott (see Abram 1996: 91–103).

The ability to be open to different possibilities about what causes distress or what provides relief or comfort is one of the pillars of good child care. As a mother learns from her baby, the baby learns about herself from her. For many babies and their mothers (and fathers or other major carers) their emergent relationships have sufficient resilience for discrepancies to be tolerated. For others, discrepancies may set very different trajectories in motion. One possibility is that inappropriate attribution of the cause of distress to defecation and faeces may produce an adverse constellation. The concretisation of pain as faeces may impair thinking about the baby as a truly psychosomatic being.

Preservation or foreclosure of developmental possibilities?

Clinical example 6.3(a)

Five-year-old Ruby was admitted to the children's ward because of chronic, medically unexplained problems defecating. Her problems had started in infancy and were now manifest as extreme distress if she felt an urge to defecate or if there were any physical interventions such as physical examination, suppositories or enemas. The intensity of her distress and the chronicity of her problems meant that a temporary colostomy was being considered. There had never been any psychiatric referral.

I was introduced to Ruby and her mother, Mrs G, by a paediatrician. I explained that my job was about helping with feelings. I was taken aback when the mother said, 'Oh, she won't understand what feelings are.'

I responded by saying to Ruby, 'I'm a doctor whose job is to try and help by understanding about upset.'

Mrs G said, 'Yes, she'll understand that.' She turned to Ruby and

---

said, 'You know when you won't have a poo, Mummy gets very upset doesn't she.'

Ruby's health and development had otherwise been within the ordinary range. She was the seventh of Mrs G's ten pregnancies, the youngest of the five surviving children. She was a delicate-looking girl who engaged readily with me. With her mother's help she was able to tell me about the upsets that had always happened if she needed a poo. Her experience was of overwhelming panic. She screamed and thrashed around, refusing to sit on the toilet. Rarely did she actually pass faeces and never into the toilet.

Agreement was reached with Mrs G. that we would attempt further non-surgical approaches. We arranged that Ruby would remain on the ward and that her mother would be with her as much as possible. The nursing staff would work alongside Mrs G administering medication and taking Ruby to the toilet. They would take over if Ruby's distress became totally incapacitating for Mrs G. In conjunction with this, I arranged to see Ruby and Mrs G for regular sessions through the week. I sought the involvement of Mr G but he did not attend because of work and family care commitments.

The nursing staff and I witnessed and experienced the intensity of distress around defecation for both Ruby and Mrs G. To be with them at these times was intensely distressing, leaving us all feeling drained. Despite the difficulties, Ruby and her mother engaged enthusiastically with us. Despite their distress they were able to allow the staff to be firm.

After two weeks, Ruby joined her mother and me for a pre-arranged consultation: Ruby was not there at the start because she had gone to the toilet with a nurse. She came in and proudly announced, 'I SAT ON THE TOILET AND HAD A POO AND I WASN'T FRIGHTENED.'

My initial exchange with Ruby and Mrs G gave me an immediate indication that disentangling their emotions and the primary and secondary influences upon them were going to be central. The foundation of any intervention was going to be an appreciation and acknowledgement of Ruby's own personal experiences rather than them being seen as derivatives of her mother's. Mrs G's responses indicated her wish to understand Ruby's emotions and communicate with her about them but her reference point was herself rather than having a truly empathic interaction with Ruby. Her engagement with clinicians in this process also demonstrated a degree of trust and ability to engage with mental processes rather than being fixed on a surgical solution.

Winnicott identified the importance of the role of a third party for a mother and baby when emotional confusions and distress arise and potentially catalyse and amplify further distress. He thought specifically about the important part fathers could play at such times (see Abram 1996: 28–30). Unfortunately it was not possible to involve Mr G. Subsequently it became apparent that this was an active resistance on his part rather than practical considerations being decisive. The ward staff and I therefore had to operate as this essential third party. The challenge was to intervene in order to create an emotional space between and for Ruby and her mother. Our task was to act as both modulators and modifiers of what they were experiencing in their world of nightmarish helplessness.

Clinical example 6.3(b)

The first therapeutic task was to see if Ruby and Mrs G could engage in constructing an alternative identity for any of the problematic elements, most particularly, Ruby's faeces. I suggested that they thought about some names for her predicament. Ruby took to this readily and it was not long before Mrs G warmed to the idea although at first she had been a bit nonplussed.

Ruby decided that her faeces would be called 'The Poo Wolf'. Poo Wolf was endowed with all the frightening characteristics of her faeces and the effects it had as it made its journey through and emergence from her. Ruby and her mother gradually expanded the story. I contributed via questions, observations and occasional prompts. As the story emerged from their ideas of fun, fear and mischief I tried to avoid interfering. I did elaborate on some points where I thought it would be useful to challenge anxieties or channel energies.

At the end of the first consultation using this approach, I asked Ruby and her mother if they could carry the story on at home. Mrs G said she would have to ask her husband to do it with Ruby. She said that he was good at that sort of thing but that she was useless.

The next consultation was the one during which Ruby was able to use the toilet for defecation for the first time. Ruby and Mrs G were excited and enthusiastic in telling me about the Poo Wolf. Father had refused to be involved. However, they had not given up. Mother decided that if father would not do it, she would have to try. They had had an uproarious time inventing a super-hero to combat Poo Wolf; they had named him 'Super Poo'. They described various scenarios in which the super-villain had lost to the super-hero, much in the style of cartoons which revolve around an unending cycle of battles through

---

which the balance always tips back to good overcoming bad. Ruby insisted on her mother repeating the cycles.

Ruby continued to be able to defecate in the toilet without fear during a two-month period of outpatient contact. Further attempts to engage the father failed. In the consultations it became apparent how profoundly Mrs G's history of miscarriages, before and after her pregnancy with Ruby, had affected her through that pregnancy and subsequently. The recounting of this did not interfere with them continuing to engage in developing 'Poo Wolf' stories further. The stories came to have a more fairy tale pattern: adversity was negotiated and 'happy ever after' became possible. I asked Mrs G if she ever read fairy tales to the children and yet again she took me by surprise. She told me that she did not read fairy tales to them because she herself found them too frightening.

It was not possible to continue Ruby's treatment so I was not able to find out if there had been consolidated progress along the developmental line 'from wetting and soiling to bladder and bowel control'. It may have only been a temporary remission – perhaps a 'flight into health' or a 'transference cure'.[6] Mrs G informed me that her husband had withdrawn his agreement to their attendance and she did not feel she could go against his wishes.

In the course of Ruby's treatment it was possible to clarify that there was preservation of developmental potential: it was ready and waiting to come into action. It was also possible to elucidate some of the initiating, maintaining and perpetuating influences. Some of these were from Ruby's internal world but major influences arose from her family. Added to this were factors within the professional context. The necessary therapeutic knowledge and clinical skills had not been available previously. Attempts to help had probably compounded a process of physicalisation rather than progression to mentalisation. The outcome of my involvement was not entirely satisfactory. I had helped to prevent unnecessary surgery but I remained concerned about the prognosis and about what else might be happening in the family.

In terms of its overall impact on me, I was left very aware of my limitations. Despite my position, experience and knowledge, and despite my demonstrable usefulness, I was left feeling powerless. This can be understood at many levels, but in the present context, the countertransferential possibilities need to be considered. Most obviously it might reflect Ruby's experience of the overwhelmingness of her body and an environment which could not hold and contain her emotions and projections sufficiently. It could also reflect Mrs G's experience of parenting particularly in context of the number of times she had not been able to carry babies through pregnancy and into the world.

My role became one of contending with and containing a sense of the enormity of the problems as they experienced them without feeling overwhelmed, contending with them without being defeated by them. I was not able to be as *helpful* as I wanted to be, but I had nevertheless been *useful*. But any need I had to *feel helpful* was my problem. This is a crucial differentiation in managing personal and countertransference pressures. Inadvertently clinicians may be driven to unhelpful activity – useless or even harmful – by the urge to do or say something to make a situation feel better when what is needed is to tolerate feelings without acting out (in) the countertransference. Winnicott also captures this in his delineation of the functions of *doing* and *being*.[7] Put succinctly, the irritated exclamation 'Don't just sit there, do something' sometimes needs to be changed round to 'Don't just do something, sit there.'

The picture I am painting is a re-emphasis of the centrality of knowing our place as professionals. Our role is circumscribed and defined by the authority accorded to us by knowledge, experience, the law **and** by the use that children, parents, other significant people in their lives and our colleagues can make of us. Our usefulness may be further circumscribed by our previous actions or those of colleagues. Patients' and parents' previous interactions may produce conscious and unconscious preconceptions about what we are and what we do. These in turn may influence our current or future usefulness. Taking account of these can be crucial particularly if a therapeutic impasse arises. Preconceptions may involve factual errors or they can be impressionistic, reflecting previous involvements and interventions.

Clinical example 6.4

Ken was eight years old when I first met him. He had been diagnosed with Hirschprung's disease[8] at eight months old. This had been operated on with apparent success but he had never achieved ordinary faecal continence; no physical explanation had been found for this. Ken was Mrs K's child from a relationship prior to her marriage to Mr K. They had five children together. Mr K had been involved and supported Mrs K at the time of Ken's initial surgery. Both parents were involved in the child psychiatric process. Generally they were cooperative with clinical staff but they came across as reserved in their manner. The impression was of needing to gain their trust rather than being able to start from a position of them having confidence in what would happen and how they would be treated.

Psychiatric referral was finally made when Ken was re-admitted to deal with a further episode of faecal impaction which required treatment with oral medication and enemas. In an early consultation

---

with Ken he drew some figures. He did this spontaneously while we were talking about school and other topics. He included a bearded figure readily identifiable as me along with some other figures (see Figure 11).

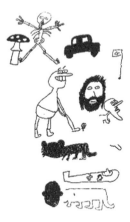

Figure 11

It was very striking how disconnected the different elements were. He did not choose to 'draw a picture' with a form and narrative of its own. The figures were sometimes incomplete and did not sit in any obvious relation to each other. The sarcophagus/Mummy near the bottom of the page did link with a school topic, but the message seemed to be about death as this also featured with the skeleton.

From the form and content I was led to wondering about how Ken thought his body parts and functions fitted together. He said he wanted to sort out his bowel problems but that he did not know when he needed a poo – he didn't get any feeling of needing to have a poo nor a sense of when it was happening. I picked this up in terms of his bottom and his head not communicating with each other. I told him what I knew about his operation as a baby and asked him what he understood about how his bowels worked. He knew some things from the school curriculum but did not appear to understand much about his own bowel. He did not seem to appreciate the connectedness between eating and pooing, digestion and waste, so I included some simple 'education' and arranged for some continuation of this by the play therapist and nurses.

In my discussion with his mother I explained about Ken's apparent lack of knowledge and understanding. It immediately emerged that

Ken's mother had not herself understood what had been done. She did not realise that the operation had been curative. She had no expectation of him ever developing bowel continence.

The admission was followed by community nurse involvement and continued psychiatric consultation. No consistent improvement occurred. Initially Mr K had been supportive and encouraging of Ken, but his ambivalence towards him became more apparent and was confirmed by Mrs K. It also became clear that there were significant problems in Mr K's treatment of his wife. She did not feel able to leave or do anything to stop what was happening. They then withdrew from treatment.[9]

As described previously, symptoms are often 'over-determined'. In Ken and Ruby's cases there were a variety of components any of which might have been considered sufficient in themselves to cause problems. In Ruby's case therapeutic engagement allowed clarification that developmental potential was preserved and there was some indication that this could be robust and resilient. In Ken's case I could not elucidate what was likely to be *reactive* as opposed to *internally self-perpetuating*. The particular constellation also contained elements of an 'antisocial tendency'.

Bottom-up organisations

Most problems relating to encopresis are not as complex as Ruby's and Ken's. Parents help their children through episodes of difficulty with little or no professional help. In other instances it may be possible to intervene briefly to capitalise on the strength and resilience of the child, parents and wider family.

Clinical example 6.5

Lee was four years old when referred by the paediatrician. Lee was the youngest of five children. The other children were all significantly older than him but close in age to each other. He was a bright boy, developing very well in every area except faecal continence: there were no anatomical or physiological abnormalities. After an initial contact on the ward he attended the clinic with his parents and siblings.

The assessment and treatment were carried out in the context of family consultations which provided opportunities to observe interactions and to gather factual information. Mr and Mrs Q were immigrants who worked very hard to establish and run their family business. They were determined to establish their children well academically and instilled a strong work ethic. They were successful in both respects and their older children were thriving. All the family were very committed and involved in Lee's care. It was very striking how pre-occupied and well-informed all family members were about Lee and his faeces. Lee himself seemed unconcerned about his bowel function.

A key piece of factual information in the background history was that two years prior to becoming pregnant with Lee, Mrs Q had been fallen pregnant but this had developed into a hydatidiform mole.[10] This potentially life-threatening condition had been treated successfully.

Gathering the family history included using a whiteboard to draw up the family tree: it was also used to note key information about people and events. The information about the hydatidiform mole arose from asking whether there had been any other pregnancies apart from those already noted for the children in the room. Mr and Mrs Q and the older children talked about what had happened and the treatment.

Over the course of three consultations, Lee had made some progress with toileting. In the clinic he was active and sometimes fully partici-pative whilst at other times distracting. He was always a focus for the rest of his family who would attend to his every wish and whim. I commented on this, mischievously but purposefully saying that he was 'The Boss'. He liked this and agreed. In order to manage the consultation better I invited him to stand on a chair at the whiteboard and help me.

Lee stood proudly with me and was delighted when I said I was going to write 'The Boss' next to his name on the family tree. He seemed to have some sense of what the family tree represented. I asked him who was 'Second Boss' and he indicated his next-to-youngest sibling. I continued this through to 'Number Seven' with Lee putting everyone in reverse order by age, ending with his father as 'Number Seven Boss'. This was a family from a highly patriarchal culture.

All through this process, the rest of the family protested that what Lee was saying was just not true. I simply pointed out that it was him saying these things, not me. I did, however, elaborate to say that things did seem to be upside down – Lee's bottom was taking charge and did not seem to want to learn its place.

At the end of the consultation, Lee's father quietly said to me that he thought they were too focused on issues relating to Lee's poo. The following consultation I heard that Lee was now using the toilet normally and no other problems had arisen. In the consultation he was more settled and less omnipotent in his ideas and interactions. No further appointments were made.

Lee's whole family had become organised around his bottom. I thought it likely that a major factor setting this pattern in motion had been Mrs Q's obstetric problems. Lee was a wanted child but one who entered the family's life with the possibility of being very dangerous. The safe pregnancy had brought him into a family which was very attentive, warm, lively and concerned but pre-occupied. This mixture appeared to have intensified the more ordinary components of anal phase development, particularly omnipotent controlling mechanisms (see Freud A. 1965: 72–5). This was enacted in family relationships such that rather than Lee striving to make progress internally with his sphincter, it had a stranglehold on the family.

A thorough paediatric assessment in conjunction with the psychiatric consultation had probably been sufficient to avoid unhelpful interventions and to free development. It would have been interesting to analyse more of the conscious and unconscious processes contributing, but this was not necessary. It is always worth holding in mind Winnicott's (1962) enigmatic and provocative statement: 'In analysis one asks: how *much* can one be allowed to do? And, by contrast, in my clinic the motto is: how *little* need be done?'

Summary and conclusions

The establishment of bodily control involves a range of processes and functions, from diffuse, generalised aspects of motor activity through to focused anatomical areas and bodily functions. In considering whole body movements and bowel movements together in a single chapter there is more than simply a play on words. Both require and involve degrees of neurological, neuromuscular and psychological maturation. Out of these developments arise the ordinary processes of socialisation.

There is a demonstrable, localisable anatomical sphincter for the bowel[11] and an analogous, non-anatomically delineated, diffuse sphincter process in relation to motor activity and attention. The key quality of a sphincter is that it can keep an orifice closed – it can prevent things getting in and getting out. In fact it is an opening, a gateway for entry and exit.

When the usual developmental trajectory in relation to motion and motions are not being followed, the possible influences need to be considered across the full breadth of biopsychosocial factors. This includes paying particular attention to the fact that the lack of ordinary socialisation can be unpleasant, annoying and inconvenient for those around the child.

This emphasises adults' responsibility to give full attention to conscious and unconscious aspects evoked or provoked in them by children. There is a profound responsibility to consider whether the environment is truly facilitating for **this** child. Is it 'good-enough' in providing a framework which the child is equipped to deal with? Might the child with attention deficit hyperactivity disorder in fact be deficient in the necessary forms of attention he requires, and hyperactively seeking a better-ordered environment for himself?

BECOMING A SPECIALIST IN NOT-KNOWING

Choose your specialist and you choose your disease (Anon 1908)

The symptoms patients suffer may not be matched by physical signs or investigatory evidence of anatomical or pathophysiological findings. Symptoms without signs constitute up to 20 per cent of general practice consultations and up to half of consultations in secondary care (National Mental Health Development Unit 2011). Defining our place as clinicians in these situations is not clear-cut. Sometimes giving assurance to patients that they are safe may be sufficient but patients must also be able to turn to doctors and other clinicians when they need reassurance. Medical science may not provide procedural answers to what a clinician should do when a patient has continuing or repeated concerns but the art of medicine requires an ability to manage these situations. The desire to find a means of communicating understanding and lack of understanding is a core clinical attribute.

The language used to describe situations where undiagnosable symptoms occur seems to need to change over time possibly because whatever terminology is used the connotations stray into the realms of moral judgementalism or dismissiveness. More recently the term 'medically unexplained symptoms' (MUS) (or 'medically unexplained physical symptoms') has come into use. It is defined as 'persistent bodily complaints for which adequate examination does not reveal sufficient explanatory structural or other specified pathology' (National Mental Health Development Unit 2011: 1). The range of severity and chronicity of impairment is extensive. When children and adolescents suffer in this way, there can be profound implications for their development and family life. Their care exemplifies the case for ensuring that paediatrics, psychiatry and psychodynamics are fully integrated.

Vanessa and Bert[1]

Clinical example 7.1(a)

Vanessa had longstanding symptoms which had been ascribed previously to urinary tract infections and respiratory tract infections. She was referred by a paediatrician who had been consulted for a further opinion. There were no concerns about her general development.

Vanessa lived some distance away so the approach used was governed by this and the available clinical resources. The process included individual consultations with Vanessa, joint meetings with her parents, separate meetings with her parents and family sessions. A key component was communication by letter.

Vanessa was eleven years old when I first saw her. Her immediate symptoms were pains in her ears and throat. She had been unwell for four years and had missed considerable schooling. Vanessa's parents were at a loss. When they saw her in pain they had to decide if the best response was to give analgesia and for her not to take part in usual activities. Alternatively did they need to proceed in expectation of the pains reducing so that rather than being off school sick, she needed their help to get across the threshold of school to face and master anxieties which might be contributing to, or causing, the physical complaints? Primarily it was her mother who had to decide. Symptoms did not only occur on school days but there was a mixture of part or full days off school and periods of extended absence. This had a major impact on the whole of family life.

The background was that the family had moved house shortly after Vanessa's birth, leaving behind a close-knit extended family and network of friends. This was an extremely difficult time for the mother. She had suffered from urinary tract infections during the pregnancy and these problems had continued in the puerperium. With upheaval and illness came a period of postnatal depression which resolved without outside intervention.

When I saw her on her own, Vanessa was amenable and pleasant. There was no suggestion of any specific problems beyond her physical complaints and the impact of these on her life. Vanessa readily engaged in the consultation but it did not develop a momentum of her spontaneously contributing or elaborating topics nor using any of the materials available for drawing or playing. I felt as though I needed to take the initiative and decided to see if 'Squiggles' would be useful.

Winnicott (1953: 108) developed the technique of using 'Squiggles' diagnostically and therapeutically. He described it as 'a game in which I first make a squiggle and [the child] turns it into something, and then he makes a squiggle and I turn it into something'. My principal teacher in child psychiatry had trained with Winnicott and took over his post when he retired: she was respectful but not idealising of his work and was highly circumspect about the use of the technique (Elmhirst 1996). I have described it as 'an unstandardised, unsystematised projective and therapeutic technique which contains the danger of telling us as much, if not more, about the *tester* as about the *tested* without either party necessarily being aware of it' (Sutton 2001a: 6). However, I did use it occasionally and sparingly.

Clinical example 7.1(b)

Vanessa took readily to the Squiggle game. As she elaborated on the squiggles I offered her, I asked if there was any story to go with the drawing. A pattern arose where the story she told came to a full stop at which there was simply 'danger'. Vanessa was not anxious in talking about this.

During my further consultations with Vanessa and her parents, I regularly found myself extremely tired. In fact, sometimes I would be struggling to stay awake let alone to attend properly and think clearly. Fully recognizing this took some time but brought about a decrease in this 'symptom'.

Reflecting on my state of mind, I thought there were two key elements. In the absence of any other identifiable variable, the improvement in my functioning provided support for the hypothesis that it was in fact a counter-transference phenomenon. Secondly, the fact that it took me some time to recognise what was happening needed understanding better. Using the countertransference was an established part of my routine clinical practice that had become dormant in me in my consultations with Vanessa. Not only was I unable simultaneously to experience and think, I had also lost the ability to register that something unusual was happening. I did not 'have it in me' or at least 'couldn't find it in myself'. It seemed to me that the challenge I faced was to try and avoid losing all sense of myself as a functioning human being and that this told me something about Vanessa's own experience.[2]

Indentifying the diagnosis

Clinical example 7.1(c)

Having reassembled myself, I took a different direction, derived from my training with Dr Sebastian Kramer.[3] I explained to Vanessa and her parents that neither I, nor the other doctors, had a good name for her illness. What we did know was that there was no indication of anything dangerous going on in her body. I suggested that as we could

---

not provide a good name, she should think of one. Vanessa was able to produce the missing diagnosis – 'Bert'.

Vanessa relished this approach and was able to play with the idea with me. I asked where Bert would live if he could not live in her ears or throat. After some consideration she spontaneously said, 'I need to find a place in my heart for him.'

I suggested that we needed to try and get to know Bert during the sessions and in letters during the gaps. We attempted to compile a life history of Bert, to work out what he might look like and even to 'introduce' him to Vanessa's still-cherished transitional object (Winnicott 1951; Holmes 2011a), Kenneth, a soft toy animal.

A sheltered life

The examples which follow are taken from some correspondence in our second year of contact.

Clinical example 7.1(d)

Dear Dr Sutton

I don't know quite what to write but I will have a go at writing Berts life fist [first] of all he was born or invented 6 years ago about when I was 7 he gave me shope [sharp] pains shooting across my chest, then later on about a year he gave me really bad pains on my tummy around my tummy around my bladder I think that's right. Then ever since he [word deleted] gave me cystitis or a bad throat and ears which where [were] very sore and he has just been doing it ever since, only now he also makes me feel very tired and weak. I get tired very easily. When he isn't giving me sore ears or throat he is playing and having fun. I think when he gives me sore ears and throat he is rebellng! From staying in one place all the time ...

Vanessa had her thirteenth birthday just after this letter and I wrote to her three weeks later.

Dear Vanessa

I'm not surprised you didn't quite know how to write about Bert, but I think you've made a very good start. I think it's a bit of a puzzle about whether he was born or whether he was invented. If he was invented maybe he didn't have two people – a Mummy and a Daddy

– who made him but only a single inventor. What do you think? I suppose if he was invented he can stay inside someone, but if he is born, he's got to get outside. No wonder he's rebelling if he reckons he's really been born and not invented! ...

Eleven days later, Vanessa replied:

Dear Dr Sutton

I think Bert was invented but I also think he thinks he was born some times like when he rebells. I don't think he knows if he was born or invented. I only know he was created either by his Mum and Dad or by a inventor or even a professor.

Bert has been rebelling a bit lately. I have been off school for a week but I am going back by the end of the week. But I have been doing some school work today I did Italian and german.

I had a lovely easter and got a lot of nice presents thank you. I went to my aunt's wedding and she had asked me to do the reading in the church. I was rather nerves about doing the reading but I managed to do it.

See you soon
Vanessa Smith

Three weeks later (1st April)

Dear Dr Sutton

I have decided that Bert was not born or invented but he was created out of on[e] of my pains. What do you think about that! I have also decided that Bert and Kenneth could probably meet, if they really try to find each other.

If they did find each other I think they would both be jealous, Kenneth because Bert knows diffrent stuff about me, like Kenneth only knows the outside of me where's Bert knows the inside of me.

This is all very confusing I know but when or if they find each other I think it will all fit into place (I hope!!)...

...Hope you had no April fools jokes?...

A week later, I responded.

Dear Vanessa

So, Bert was neither born nor invented but created out of one of your pains! What on earth does a creature like that look like? This is going to be extremely important to know because how on earth would Kenneth know what to look for if he did decide to go in search of him?

The problem is that neither you, me, your Mum and Dad, nor any of the doctors in the hospital have ever actually seen him – so, how can we get a proper description? We are going to have to work on what the police would call 'an artist's impression'. It's more difficult for us though because we've only got your inside-feelings to go on and not your eye-sight or mine. I'd like you to write down what different bits of him feel like and then draw a picture of him. By the way, how do you know it's a 'he' not a 'she'?

It's also clear that we mustn't rush Bert and Kenneth into a meeting – it sounds like they both want you all to themselves – one knows you inside: one knows you outside: it's going to take time for them to learn that they can both know you inside-out without losing you to anyone else. They are going to have to learn this from you and it's going to take time. So, they mustn't meet yet otherwise there will be fireworks! You'll need to work out how to teach them that it's safe to share (it might even be fun): can you start writing about it?

Best wishes,

Doctor Sutton

Ups and downs

The pattern was one of fluctuating symptoms but with an overall sense of less severe recurrences and overall progress. Bert was a slippery character, difficult to pin down. In the spirit of characterising and locating him, I posed the question, 'Where is Bert when he's not living in your throat or ears?'

The reply came by letter.

Clinical example 7.1(e)

Dear Dr Sutton

I have decided that Bert should live in my big toe. I don't know why but it just seems to be a good place for him to go. Because if he does turn nasty all he could do is make me stub my toe or make me break my toe, it is quite small so he can't get into mischief but also quite big in some ways so he will have enough room to play in.

Yesterday we put up the Christmas tree it looks very nice.

On Friday night I got the results from my music exam I passed with honours I got 87% out of 100%. I hope you like your Christmas card. I picked it myself...

In my reply, I commented on the idea of Bert needing a place that was big enough, but not so big that he felt lonely or lost. I suggested we could try and make friends with him.

Vanessa arrived for her next consultation on crutches. There had been an accident. She had dropped a mirror on her left foot. Walking awkwardly as a result, she had slipped, badly sprained her ankle hence the crutches. Subsequently it was decided that she needed her ankle to be put in a plaster cast. This setback needed careful handling to avoid excessive caution which might lead to unhelpful medical activity. The tightrope to be walked was to neither deny the pain of the identifiable injury or unhelpfully to 'feed' the psychopathology driving her chronic difficulties. We had the following exchange of letters.

Dear Dr Sutton

Alfred has been in a very good mood recently. My ears and throat don't hurt that much recently but my foot isn't any better. I have had my foot in a pot for 2 weeks. I got it off on Monday. My foot is still very sore and swollen, I am still on crutches. I am also having physiotherapy at the moment (that is quite painful).

So really Bert is being rather good at the moment, so is Kenneth.

I have been to school....

I replied:

Dear Vanessa

I'm sorry to hear your foot is still hurting and that physio is difficult. Still, it seems to have kept Bert in one place, trapped underneath the plaster-cast. But I do feel sad for him trapped down there. You say he's been 'good'. I don't really think it's being 'good' or 'bad'. If you think about it, it must be pretty difficult being all on your own, in the dark with nobody who even knows what you look like let alone how you're feeling. Kenneth has a much easier life.

I think he needs someone to take proper notice of him and to go to great lengths to get to know him properly – just like Kenneth has. So, it's down to you Vanessa. You've got to be his 'Super-Hero', discovering him, shining some light on to him, then he can be seen and known. I reckon he'll be frightened at first then he'll find it a relief. I even have a suspicion that he might turn out to be something like Kenneth – maybe even his long-lost twin.

So, Vanessa let's have the story of 'Vanessa the Intrepid Explorer seeks and finds Bert'. I think it will need to be a long story and probably needs words and pictures. Can you try and make a start on it before we next meet?......

Best wishes

Doctor Sutton

The conflicts between being known and not-known and being both interested in the unknown and fearful of it represent a point for the potential emergence of a 'false self'. The 'true self' is an outward expression of an inner need which has to assert itself. This assertion will be amplified unless the need is met more closely or unless 'obliterating' mechanisms are activated. The 'false self' accommodates to the not-good-enough environment to manage by a form of 'double bluff' – splitting off in the sense of having failed and over-capitalising on both the successful part of the environment and on the ego strengths which make this possible. This component of the 'true self' then becomes fixated, stuck in this position of 'not having it in itself to manage' rather than this being influenced by the overall maturational processes. The see-saw of asserting need and denying or hiding it can become enacted around bodily experiences.

It is also important to disentangle whether or not symptoms have symbolic significance. It was likely that dropping the mirror on to her foot was a manifestation of unconscious conflicts. However, I saw the subsequent processes as the consequence of the dysfunction associated directly with the pain and need to adapt rather than being further primary effects of those conflicts. As Freud may have said, 'Sometimes a cigar is just a cigar'.[4] The injury did have the potential to become incorporated into the overall process, a further part of the illness narrative. It could be 'seized upon' by regressive forces including those which exploit the potential for experiencing power in relationships.

The achievement of neurosis

Despite intermittent periods of illness, Vanessa was able to maintain contact with her friends and regain considerable ground academically. Her attainments were slightly behind her peers: school attributed this to her extended absences. However, I thought she had unrecognised specific difficulties in reading and writing. Formal assessment confirmed this and personal tutoring helped.

When she was 16, there was an episode of severe and sudden onset of new symptoms of a different quality. These resulted in neurological investigations. Close liaison with her parents, her paediatrician and a neurologist ensured that these investigations did not extend beyond necessity and usefulness.

Over a few weeks, I was able to disentangle answers to the questions 'Why now?' and 'Why these symptoms?'

Clinical example 7.1(f)

Vanessa had been on a trip with her mother and grandmother when she suddenly experienced frighteningly intense dizziness.

Her grandmother had recently experienced an acute psychological trauma. On this trip the grandmother was returning, for the first time, to a place with particular associations to it. Vanessa had momentarily lost sight of her grandmother. That was when her physical symptoms had struck. The specific symptoms related both to the nature of the grandmother's trauma and to the immediate situation.

I gathered a very detailed history from Vanessa about the episode. At the point of experiencing the symptoms Vanessa was not conscious of any links between immediate and past events, nor their significance to herself and in her relationships. We analysed the episode contextualising it in the overall process of her therapy which led to the above formulation. It made sense of why she had experienced **these** symptoms at **this** point.

Direct therapeutic gain followed from this process.

The diffuse experience of 'dangerousness' which crystallised in the Squiggle game and was present in her usual physical symptoms had been replaced by a more focused process for which we could find words. This was a very different constellation from the way problems had previously presented. In contrast to the pattern of diffuse symptoms in her previous psychosomatic presentations, it was a definable *dissociative (conversion) illness* [F44] episode as defined in the ICD–10 (WHO 2007).

The underlying structures and defence mechanisms required to produce the diffuse experience as opposed to the dissociative are very different. In the former, the mechanisms obliterate experience, whilst in the latter they 'manage' the internal conflict, negotiating the demands of both external reality and internal unconscious phantasy. Developmentally the first belongs to an earlier stage of life – Vanessa had achieved the ability to have a neurosis.

Developmental challenge and developmental gain

After her final year of secondary education, at the age of 18 Vanessa wrote to me after a few months without any intervening correspondence.

Clinical example 7.1(g)

Dear Dr Sutton

Why is it that when you should be happy and care free that almost depression glides over your whole life?

I have got my results and now I am at the university of my choice, to do the course I have picked. I have a fantastic boyfriend and some brilliant mates. I am working and therefore earning money with great employers.

But it seems as if there is something missing. I'm on autopilot and it seems like I'm not living my own life, physically it does with the tiredness after working for five hours, but mentally it is somebody else doing it. It's not me. I guess the truth is it's Bert, which makes me realise that I will be alright in a few days, and my bubbly personality will shine but in the mean time I will continue to operate under a dark cloud.

The strongest feeling inside me at the moment is to escape, go away, think and most importantly relax, which I feel physically I haven't done in months, what with school, then work.

The last I wrote to you I spoke about a feeling of control, well that has gone for the moment. I lost hold of it and am now dreaming about retrieving it.

I am at works becon [beck and] call and the rest of the time I have to divide between Dave (my boyfriend) and my mates. Where am I supposed to find time to myself? ...

Whilst writing this letter I am listening to the Alanis Morrisette album, I don't know if you have ever heard any of her but personally I believe the lyrics are surprisingly relevant in reality and life as I am finding it. In one song called Perfect some of the lyrics are

[']Don't forget to keep that smile on your face. What's the problem ...why are you crying?[']

I guess they apply to most people. I know I will get through this bleak period as I have survived the last years of my life. But hey a smile doesn't have to be present ['pleasant' crossed out] constantly on my face.

It's wired [weird?] I can hardly remember what I wrote at the begin[n]ing of this letter. But what I do know is that I feel better for writing. In case you hadn't realised this is one of the first times I have been absolutely honest about my feelings to you. And as Bob Dylan sang in the first few lines of all along the watch tower

[']There must be some way out of here

There's too much confusion

I can't get no relief...[']

I replied:

Dear Vanessa

It was lovely to receive your letter. That may sound a bit strange when it was about feeling sad and empty. But it was a beautiful letter because of how clearly you explained what it is you are struggling with and how you keep hope alive at the same time as these other feelings – knowing 'Bert' is part of you even if it feels like someone else taking you over.

Congratulations on your university place. I was wondering if you might like to meet once more, before you start there. That would give us a chance to talk about your letter and to think a bit about the future …

Vanessa replied:

Dear Dr Sutton

The sadness that [was] prevalent through my last letter is gradually disappearing as I knew it would. However this only began when I was honest with myself and to my parents – I'm not sure whether I want to go to university or not.

At the moment there are plenty of choices however there are only two main ones. Go to university or train as a medical technician which is something I considered a while back.

However I only have a couple of weeks to decide!!

I think it would be a good idea to meet up again …

Vanessa

In the past Vanessa's difficulty in making decisions had become part of the family's folk lore. I later came to recognise obsessional mechanisms featured in all psychosomatic presentations. However, by the time we met, Vanessa had decided on a clear course of action. She was not going to go university and was confident about what she was going to do instead.

Vanessa eloquently explained that she had set her plans to fit with what she felt other people expected of her – who they thought she was (or perhaps who she thought they thought she was). She had known for a long time that this was how she lived her life, but now she felt able to stand up to this part *of herself*. Vanessa was able to *find it in herself* to do this. Now she could let it be known what her own desires were, and simultaneously tolerate in her relationships the experience of taking other people by surprise by doing this. She had been a specialist in making 'not-known' a fundamentally important part of herself. But it was no longer forcing itself to her attention by playing hide and seek in her body. Now she could tolerate this being a known and readily recognised part of herself and still feel safe.

Vanessa felt anxious but was filled with a pleasurable anticipation of what the future held. What previously emerged in her symptoms could belong to her fully, integrated into her emotional life. She no longer had any physical symptoms.

Classification in relation to psychoanalytic principles

The diagnostic issues for Vanessa have been described in a way which gives a developmental perspective to psychiatric classification. Psychiatrically she moved from 'MUS' through dissociative (conversion) disorder to depression. This developmental perspective can be given 'psychodynamic flesh' which can assist in formulating trajectories, progressions and regressions which can help organise our clinical thinking and research.

Anna Freud (1970) defined a complementary pair of classificatory systems of childhood patterns of symptom presentation. She called these:

- *Symptomatology Proper*: the underlying intra psychic constellations which produce manifest problems.
- *Other Signs of Disturbance:* approaches classification by travelling in the reverse direction, 'from surface signs...to whichever upheaval, involvement or failure may be responsible for them'.

Individually, symptoms and signs may be non-specific but linking manifest symptoms and unconscious mental processes 'draw[s] the diagnostician's contribution away from the child's [manifest] pathology and to return it instead to an assessment of his developmental status and the picture of his total personality'. Using this dual approach can lead to groupings which can be differentiated into discrete constellations by a cross-referencing of the two systems. Freud believed this would mean children could be understood in the breadth of their development **and** in the immediate context of relationships, expectations and other environmental influences. A corollary is that greater diagnostic accuracy can be achieved in terms of the balance of internal or external factors. Freud proposed that ultimately this would provide a route through which appropriate matching of disorder and therapy could be achieved, and through which prognostic accuracy may be improved.

Under '*Other Signs of Disturbance*', Freud grouped: 'Aches and pains (psychosomatic, hysterical, hypochondriacal)' to indicate their superficial homogeneity as perceived by others and as consciously experienced by the individual herself. Within the class of '*Symptomatology Proper*' she described two (out of six) groupings where physical symptoms may dominate: '1. Symptoms resulting from initial nondifferentiation between somatic and psychological processes [i.e.] psychosomatic presentations... 6. Symptoms resulting from undefended regressions [i.e.] infantilisms and pseudodebility.' The first reflects foreclosure, the latter regression. Physical symptoms may also present as conversion neurosis which requires greater maturity of ego development but this represents a very different constellation with symptom formation emerging as a 'compromise' between id and ego-functioning (Freud's Group 2).

Vanessa illustrates developmental progression in line with Freud's classificatory system. In terms of *'Symptomatology Proper'*, Vanessa moved through from Freud's Group 1 (a psychosomatic presentation) to Group 2 (hysterical conversion neurosis). Subsequently she presented with depressed mood in the absence of physical symptoms, Freud's Group 4 (symptoms resulting from changes in the libido economy or direction of cathexis).

Further psychodynamic considerations

At the root of the problems being considered is whether mechanisms emerge which minimise the adverse consequences of suffering. Some of these mechanisms reside with the inherent developmental potential; others reside within those providing care.

The eminent scientist Patrick Wall wrote the book *Pain: the science of suffering* whilst living with terminal cancer. He stated 'Coping is not ignoring. In fact, it is the opposite ... pain persists but no longer demands emergency responses. It is not a catastrophe signalling impending annihilation ... Coping is the beginning of a series of steps that give a sense of understanding and a type of control' (Wall 1999: 101). Although MUS is not life-threatening, the psychodynamic issues involved are comparable, and symptom formation indicates a failure in this form of coping. 'Danger' paradoxically registers and is obliterated – what arises is a bodily state of 'not-right-ness' dissociated from meaning and emotion.

Gaps and spaces

Life has to be lived without ever being fully equipped to communicate about it. Children need treating but we cannot know them until we have found out about them: somehow we have to cope by piecing together the ideas we do have and allowing that it may be difficult to justify fully the basis for our next thought or action. The process is iterative and reflective, striking a balance between being open to the possibility of error whilst avoiding ruminative self-disqualification.

The psychoanalyst McDougall (1989) described the predicament of patients with psychosomatic problems in ways that resonate with Wall's sense of 'coping function'. From work with Vanessa and further work with children and adolescents to be described in this chapter and Chapters 8 and 9 the issues of tolerating states of 'not-knowing' or 'not-being-known' became central. Infant-states which in psychical terms may have been described as catastrophic had to be understood as even worse than life-threatening – in fact, as a fate worse than death.

The possible alternative states under consideration have a form which is binary, as described in the psychodynamics of safety (Chapter 5). They are preverbal in origin and have not been brought under the containing, understanding and communicating influence of language and intellect. Further, the use of the physical is the means both of contending with and defending against such mental states.

Understanding the difference between a gap and a space can help us get our minds round this. *Gap*: unfilled space or interval, blank, *break* in *continuity'* [author's italics]; *space*: continuous extension viewed with or without reference to the existence of objects within it' (Concise Oxford Dictionary 1982). O'Shaughnessy (1964) proposed the concept of the *absent object* to capture the idea that a baby who fails to experience a sense of relief or safety because a carer is not actually present instead experiences her as present in a persecutory form because of relief not being obtained. In the type of psychosomatic presentation I have described, instead of the experience of the absent object, the body or a part or function of the body appears to serve as a gap-filler, as if it is the other. But it cannot *not* be 'of the self'. There is a failure to develop adequately what Winnicott (1951) came to call the 'transitional space'[6] – a space where experience can be explored without fear *for* or *of* the objects within it. Kenneth, Vanessa's transitional object, did not manage fully or consistently to carry her through or tolerate a sense of discontinuity in the gap between awareness of need and finding a good-enough response. She remained with her sense of 'wrongness' located in her body.

Drawing a blank

Clinical example 7.2

Siobhan was ten years old and had significant problems with MUS. Her therapists had been trying to encourage her to tell them more about her problems – she thought she was explaining very clearly that her physical symptoms were her problems and that she was giving complete responses to their questions. They gave her some paper and pencils to take home with her to see if she would be able to write about her 'problems'. The next appointment time only her mother attended. She handed over a letter from Siobhan and some other paper. The letter said:

I apologise if you think I'm being rude but I do not like coming only because it does not help ... I have given you back the papers just as they were because I feel blank! But there is one picture I drew, <u>well</u> splashed and it was another feeling of <u>Anger!</u> You do not make me feel any better by asking me questions? – I'm still scared you've not made it go away!

Save me. Help me! I'm not HAPPY. Grrrrrrr!

Yours angrily

Siobhan

P.S. I feel weak, tired, ill, I'm hungry only because I can never taste food. I find it difficult to breathe, I get tired easily, I also cry easily and I'm fed up! And I swear I'm not going against you in any way! I [k]now your trying to make me better but it's just <u>not</u> working.

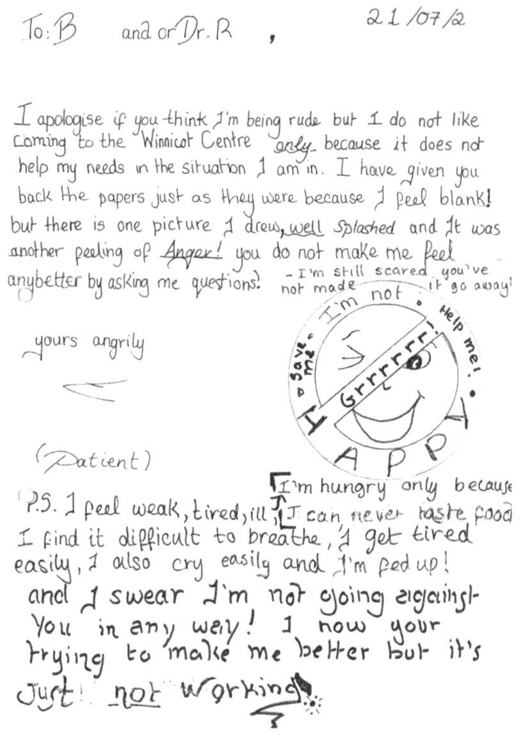

Figure 12

Siobhan speaks eloquently about a blank – a gap – as what needed to be understood alongside problems of physical symptoms. She certainly knew her feelings, and articulated them, something which is often talked of as a fundamental 'ability gap' in these forms of presentation (see *alexythymia* in Chapter 8). She wanted to be cooperative and polite. She was frustrated at the lack of an empathic response even though the therapists were kind and wanted to be helpful. She experienced an 'empathy gap' in them.

Constructing stories and playing with ideas is one way of trying to articulate and give expression to those aspects of life which are always just beyond grasping precisely: there has to be an 'as if' quality – 'as if' as pretence but also 'as if...' in the way it has come to be used particularly by adolescents (of many ages) to deny that such events could ever really happen. But to be therapeutically useful practitioners have to support the child in knowing that this gap in knowing themselves as separate can be a place where other things can be safely found. The moment of a sense of catastrophic loss is not forever.

So, who is 'Bert'?

Winnicott's constructs of the 'true self' and 'false self' describe the internal processes which may flow from very early disruptions to the experience of the external world as dependable in a form which the infant ego can cope with (see Abram 1996: 277–81). They were actually presaged by Groddeck (1920) in his formulation of the 'It'. In *The meaning of illness* Groddeck (1925) argues illness symptoms simultaneously express a striving for health. The following extract captures the spirit of the correspondence between Vanessa and I and the nature of 'Bert':

> Yet the person who does the interpreting should no longer be the physician: only the patient himself can supply the necessary information about his It and its intentions and activities. For every It has its own thought processes and ideas concerning symbolic meanings. The role of the therapist is restricted to that of making the recalcitrant It talk and even more significantly, being as open as possible in order to allow the patient's It the least possible excuse for mistrusting him.
>
> (Groddeck 1925: 101).

Vanessa and I never did get a very clear picture of Bert. We knew when he was around and certainly understood when and how he made his presence felt. A formal psychotherapy or psychoanalysis might have given a more complete answer. However, I think Bert can be understood as an encapsulated expression of Groddeck's 'It' or Winnicott's 'true self'. His characteristics reflect the failure to achieve a state in which the elements he represents could find a manageable place in the transitional space. These had not been fully contained and processed by Vanessa and her mother. Instead, these elements remained in a form which needed to be expressed and met in the arena of the body and its care rather than progressing through to symbolic expression.

Bert is the manifestation both of need which must be expressed and the defence against awareness of the arousal and threat experienced in that state.

At that earliest time of their life together, Vanessa's mother was struggling with depression and social isolation and had had chronic urinary tract symptoms. The emergence of symptoms which were diagnosed as urinary tract infection had provided a rendezvous point and a link for mother and daughter. They established a form of continuity but contributed to fixation through identifications which obliterated their separateness.

Bert's 'creation' in the therapeutic relationship was an attempt to bring him into the *transitional space*, where the most dreadful things can be done and experienced in safety. Ultimately, instead of a physical experience of pain, Bert became an emotional state which could be known as part of herself rather than living an autonomous life inside her. In addition, he became a part of her which needed to be accommodated and which could be adapted to without her believing he was going to rule her life forever.

Summary and conclusions

The detailed examination of my countertransference response and my failure to be able to manage it properly re-connected me with my training and clinical experience. From this I developed a new understanding which could be incorporated into the key relationships around Vanessa. Her parents were able to have confidence in my 'peculiar' practice through observing that it clearly resonated in some distinct way with what Vanessa needed and through it being demonstrably part of an integrated psychosomatic approach. Vanessa's paediatrician and I occupied an important space for them: I wonder if we perhaps represented transferentially the grandparental couples who were not available during the pregnancy and puerperium with Vanessa.

The approach advocated in this chapter and the following two is largely consistent with the approach recommended by the National Mental Health Development Unit (2011). Both emphasise the role of acceptance and continuity of care:

> People want to be taken seriously – show you believe them… Doctors can make a difference to the patient's well-being even when their symptoms are unexplained… Sometimes the only 'therapy' needed may be the strength of your doctor–patient relationship – continuity of care and the long-term relationship helps.
>
> (NMHDU 2011)

This contrasts with approaches which see the problem as being 'fed' if a focus remains on the presenting symptoms.

Detailed examination of the NMHDU document demonstrates the complexity of trying to work with language of any kind. What does 'strength of your doctor–patient relationship' mean – people may have a very strong relationship without this necessarily being beneficial. It is possible for doctors and patients to engage in a collusive mutuality of beliefs which are based on them being 'of the same mind' and to split off any challenge or doubts into an alternative frame of reference. There are some other subtle distinctions of profound importance in the document's wording. What does 'be pre-emptively reassuring' mean? A doctor may give *reassurance* without the patient ever being *assured* – what is likely to be more significant is exploring the fact of the patient's inability to feel assured rather than simply repeating the same thing or the same thing in different words. 'Be open about your uncertainty yet reassuring that a *serious* cause is unlikely, but stress that you will keep an open mind' [my italics] does not properly acknowledge that the impact on the patient's life (and of those close to them) can be extremely *serious* despite not being *dangerous*. Even the use of the word 'medically' inadvertently rejects the place of psychiatry or 'psychological medicine' in medicine. Perhaps the acronym derived from using the term *physically unexplained symptoms* (PUS) would convey the medical science *and* the experience better but even this would in all likelihood become infected with the same problems!

An important part of the answer lies in understanding transference and avoiding acting out in the countertransference. Psychoanalytic theory helps us understand the responses elicited in us as clinicians by this complex group of problems. From this we are better placed to manage our clinical actions to demonstrate implicitly and explicitly that we are dealing with states that relate to intense fear and that keep themselves beyond neat identification and formulation. From this we can maintain a state of proper clinical vigilance and plan better clinical management, avoiding unnecessary action whilst ensuring necessary action. 'Watchful waiting' and actively remaining clinically active demonstrates that we understand the general risks in life, the sense of risk for the patient and her parents and that managing uncertainty *with* them is developmental therapy . This is pursued further in the next chapter.

8

PRACTISING AS A SPECIALIST
IN NOT-KNOWING

Learning is an affront to omnipotence.[1]

Some children with medically unexplained symptoms are severely disabled. There can be considerable disruption to their lives and those of other family members. They may experience considerable suffering in their illnesses and in some of the responses the condition elicits. They can also place considerable demands on medical, nursing and other health services.

When a suggestion of referral for psychiatric assessment is made it may be only accepted reluctantly or even rejected. Resistance may arise for a variety of reasons and come from any of the parties involved, patient, parent or professional. From the perspective of patients and parents, suggesting psychiatric involvement can feel like a denial that there is a problem. Children may think they are being told they are imagining things. Parents may feel their experiences of being with their child's debility and pain are being brushed aside or denied. There may be fear that a *serious*, i.e. physically dangerous, illness is being, or will be, missed.

Sometimes doctors do deny that there is 'real' pain or loss of function (see *Clinical example 5.2*). It may be viewed as a manipulative interaction, a pretence through which children rule their parents who in turn may be viewed as ineffectual in not standing up to their child. Professionals may fear that they are 'missing something' or failing if they cannot solve the problem. The process can become a denial of 'not-knowing' and an unwitting enactment of omnipotent phantasies. Prejudice or prior experience may mean they do not have confidence in the services they can call upon. Some doctors may take a position that they have done all they can or should by establishing a 'diagnosis' – MUS. They may wish simply to 'refer on', discharging the patient and any responsibility towards her, leaving child and parents in fear and trepidation of the child's physical safety in the hands of 'psychs' without understanding of 'somas'.

The recommendation for psychiatric involvement is regularly presented as if a definitive diagnosis has been made, i.e. 'It's *psychological*'. In fact, what is being delineated is twofold. Firstly, that the cause of the child's symptoms is not understood. Secondly, that further investigation is most appropriately pursued in the realm of the patient's mental life and relationships. The framework presented in Chapter 7 provides structures to assist in orientating the developmental and interpersonal factors involved. In this chapter more detailed consideration is given to intrapsychic and countertransference factors which should inform general case management.

Some further considerations from psychoanalytic theory

The meaning of illness

Groddeck (1925: 197) developed some of the original psychoanalytic formulations relating to physical symptoms and accorded a central position to his concept of 'The It': 'The It – or may we call it the vital force, the self, the organism…'. This is an ill-defined construct which attempts to capture an underlying psychosomatic constellation which is the result and expression of the essential unity of physical (including genetic) and psychological processes. These have the potential to unfold with a momentum of their own whilst being shaped in complex ways by influences arising both from within the self and from external forces. Groddeck's formulation is useful in conceptualising the way in which a momentum of changing form and structure arises through existence and interaction. One form which emerges may be called 'illness'. It is created by 'this It, about which we know nothing and of which we shall never recognise more than its outward forms, [which] tries to express something by illness; to be ill has to mean something' (Groddeck 1925: 197). In Groddeck's terms, when a person is ill, his resources have been stretched beyond capability and the resultant presentation is the It's attempt to deal with this state of affairs. The corollary is that illness may contain an inherent striving towards a *better state* even if that state appears to be completely dysfunctional to the physician. In consequence, clinicians must understand the patient sufficiently to realise that they represent a threat to their patients by striving to alter this 'dysfunctional' state. Groddeck summarises this as 'The role of the therapist is restricted to that of making the recalcitrant It talk and, even more significantly, being as open as possible in order to allow the patient's It the least possible excuse for mistrusting him' (Groddeck 1925: 201).

Words and feelings: success and failure of integration

Success: metaphorically speaking

Ella Freeman Sharpe investigated the relationship between physical experience, emotional experience and language through an examination of metaphor. She viewed metaphor as essential to emotional and cognitive development: 'The intellectual life of man is only possible through the development of metaphor' (Sharpe 1940: 155). She summarised her position:

1 Metaphor evolves alongside the control of the bodily orifices. Emotions which originally accompanied bodily discharge find substitute channels and materials.

2 Spontaneous metaphor [is] an epitome of a forgotten experience ... a present-day psychical condition which is based upon an original psycho-physical experience.

3 In metaphor ... the repressed psycho-physical experiences have found the verbal images in the pre-conscious that express them. ... The person who speaks vitally in metaphor *knows*, but does not know in consciousness what he knows unconsciously.

4 An examination of metaphors used by patients reveals ... a preponderance of images based upon experiences of the pre-genital stages ...

5 They reveal something of the early incorporated environment.

6 Metaphor gives information concerning instinctual tension... (Sharpe 1940: 168).

The successful development of metaphor integrates and differentiates physical and emotional experience such that both an internal and an interpersonal dialogue can occur. It operates in *transitional zones* bringing greater likelihood of symptomatic experience being appreciated even if not completely understood. Vanessa's Bert (Chapter 7) can be considered a form of metaphor. The application of any diagnostic term may have usefulness in this way, giving an area of good-enough communication. Again, Groddeck (1925: 201) leads in the same direction: 'all this and more needs to be taken into account if one wants to get the meaning of this illness approximately right'.

Failure: metaphorically speaking

A commonly recognised feature in patients with psychosomatic problems is an apparent inability to communicate about emotions. The term *alexythymia* (also spelt alexithymia) was coined to capture this phenomenon (Nemiah and Sifneos 1970). Lask and Fosson (1989) present it as an inability to express emotions in words.

McDougall (1989: 52) observed: 'Words are remarkable containers of feeling and may prevent highly charged emotional experiences from seeking immediate discharge through the soma or release in action' but that in psychoanalytic treatment with people with psychosomatic difficulties 'it may happen that, because of certain ways of mental functioning, the emotional impact of the external world ... is excluded not only from consciousness, but also from the symbolic chain of meaningful psychic representations' (p. 163). For such people, when conflict or turbulence in the internal world reaches a certain threshold, physical symptoms will emerge because they have a restricted capacity to find or create a space inside themselves, or in relationships, for the use of language as a modulating or modifying influence.

If we listen, the body communicates that something is not right and sounds an alarm. It does not have a vocabulary beyond its physiology and anatomy. 'Not functioning or functioning' and 'locating' are the limits of this. The patient's maturational achievements allow them to tell us about this; however the problem is not one of *alexythymia* as described above. Where the observer expects emotions to be, there is a gap. As clinicians we have to recognise that our usual expectation or aspiration that language and intellect can provide us with precision must fail if we are to understand what needs to be understood. There is a 'nameless dread' (Bion 1957). 'Being there' and 'functioning' are the roles that are needed. Confirmation is needed that life continues despite overwhelmed-ness being experienced. Repeated *containment* and *holding* through these experiences can confirm that a fate worse than not existing has not happened.

Synthesis in theory and practice

The task in Vanessa's therapy and development was to facilitate the establishment of more robust transitional mechanisms. These would provide an essential buffer to absorb excessive environmental buffeting. In the absence of this achievement such stimuli could only result in physical symptoms and a sense of 'wrongness' and danger without other content: her 'proto- defences' obliterated other emotional or cognitive experience. 'Bert', the diagnostic identity we constructed, served to identify that we knew a little of who or what we were talking about at the same time as acknowledging that we did not know it all. Despite recognising that words failed in many ways, we could still share an experience that it was worth carrying on communicating. Out of this, Vanessa and I developed a shared language and constructed a story which captured the sense of 'self and other' with continuities of being that were sufficient for developmental progress to occur.

This formulation provides a link in theory and practice, between the formulations of Groddeck, Anna Freud, McDougall and Sharpe (and implicitly links with Winnicott's (1953) formulations in the same arena).

Working in and through the countertransference

Kraemer and Loader (1995: 937) highlighted the primary importance of the countertransference for patients with psychosomatic problems: 'What is often more important in coming to a conclusion about psychosomatic disorder is not so much the state of mind of the patient as that of the doctor.' McDougall (1989: 91) described how this manifested in her clinical work: 'As time went on, some of these patients made me feel paralyzed in my analytic functioning. I could neither help them to become more alive nor lead them to terminate analysis. The affectless quality of certain sessions made me feel weary, and I would find my attention wandering. In addition, their spectacular lack of progress made me feel guilty.' The therapist has to work on themselves.

The enemy within and without

The challenge I faced with this area of work was to maintain myself as an alive, thinking person who could contain states of not-knowingness whilst countering pressures towards obliteration of experience. This formulation became encapsulated in the phrase 'becoming a specialist in not-knowing'. The following material from other clinical work conducted subsequently underlines this and elucidates further dynamics of psychosomatic presentations, particularly those manifest in countertransference processes.

Heather

Clinical example 8.1(a)

When Heather was 11 years old she became acutely ill and diabetes mellitus was diagnosed. During a brief admission, her initial treatment regime was established. Her parents had just separated after long-standing marital problems and Heather and her mother and siblings moved to a different part of the country.

Heather's diabetes was described as 'brittle'. Her blood glucose fluctuations did not settle into a safe pattern manageable with a standard treatment regime. At times her blood sugar levels became so seriously disrupted that she had episodes of unconsciousness: during some of these there were reports of probable convulsions. After moving house it was not easy for Heather to find her feet in the new neighbourhood. At school, the demands of academic work were not a problem, but peer relationships were difficult. This was manifest as a lack of ease in relationships and a sense of 'apart-ness' rather than hostility, i.e. there was internal discomfort rather than interpersonal conflict.

Life-threatening difficulties led to referral to my paediatric colleagues and I when Heather was 13 years old. After what had appeared to be a minor gastrointestinal upset, vomiting persisted. The pattern was described as 'effortless vomiting'. There was no identifiable physical pathology or mechanisms which could be considered 'deliberate' on the part of Heather. In conjunction with her brittle diabetes, this was potentially a life-threatening crisis since the ability to maintain stable glucose and blood electrolyte levels was severely compromised. This acute presentation became chronic. She was referred for a second opinion and consideration of joint management by myself and paediatric nursing and medical colleagues on a general paediatric ward.

Heather's ward management was complicated from both the physical and psychological point of view. She could be challenging in ways which

---

at times felt 'spirited' when striving to assert herself in order to prevent the 'wrong' thing happening; at other times it could feel oppositional or desperate, or perhaps both, the latter, or all three simultaneously.

I provided twice-weekly individual sessions with Heather, weekly individual joint consultations with Heather and her mother and consistent close liaison with the nursing and medical team. This was far removed from the 'treatment of choice'. My view was that each role should have been carried out by a separate practitioner but more suitable alternative resources were not available.

Heather engaged in her treatment but was rarely able to initiate conversations in her individual psychotherapy. Her sessions needed to take place in her room on the ward due to practical constraints on clinical space. This was added to, at times, by the seriousness of her physical condition. On entering her room, the assault on my senses of the smell of vomit was appalling. Being in the room hearing and seeing her vomiting, smelling the stench could be dreadful. Maintaining a psychotherapeutic availability presented the usual challenges described for psychosomatic presentations although the combined effect of her symptoms and signs was probably equivalent to a dose of smelling salts.

There were fluctuations in Heather's symptoms during my contact with her (in excess of five years), but there was never a sense of fundamental progress. It was difficult sometimes to hold on to the idea that there really was a way to be of use by being 'a doctor who helps by understanding about upsets'. Heather and her mother did find benefit from the approach even though the physical symptoms persisted to an incapacitating degree. At one point she was admitted to a psychiatric unit specialising in eating disorders. The formulations of Heather's problems by that unit and myself did differ significantly but I felt a change was called for given my inability to help her make progress and their more extensive resources. She returned to my care again later.

Ultimately I felt I was able to identify significant historical and ongoing issues from a psychodynamic perspective that were significant contributors to the development of *a* disorder, even if they did not help specify why it was *this* disorder.

Watching the detectives

Clinical example 8.1(b)

One morning, a few months into the contact with Heather, I was walking back down the ward after seeing Heather for a psychotherapy session, when I found myself thinking about the fictional television detective, Columbo.[3] Not only was I thinking about him, I felt as if I *was* him, walking in the same slouched and pre-occupied manner. It was not a programme I had been particularly interested in nor watched more than occasionally many years previously, so it was perhaps more readily possible to recognise that something 'had got into me', i.e. it was a countertransference phenomenon.

There was nothing specifically identifiable from the session's content leading to this association arising, so I reflected more widely. Columbo has a particular style. He presents himself in his whole demeanour as unkempt and ramshackle. His manner with potential suspects is one of perpetual puzzlement and of being incapable of making sense of anything. His persona is of being someone for whom only questions arise, not answers. Yet, out of this scenario, somehow, he creates a situation in which the culprits are lulled into errors that make their guilt undeniable. In essence, he makes an art of being the embodiment of 'not-knowing and not-being-capable-of-becoming-knowing'. As a specialist in 'not-knowing', he enacts an impotent, denigrated object. This in turn intensifies the other half of this split in the murderer – omnipotence and invulnerability. The culprit, in the hold of these powerful projective processes, enacts this and lets their guard slip. Inevitably they enact their phantasised omnipotence, make mistakes and 'give themselves away'.

Columbo's approach has direct comparisons with that advocated by Groddeck:

> Yet the person who does the interpreting should no longer be the physician; only the patient himself can supply the necessary information about his It and its intentions and activities. ... The role of the therapist is restricted to that of making the recalcitrant It talk and, even more significantly, being as open as possible in order to allow the patient's It the least possible excuse for mistrusting him.
>
> (Groddeck 1925: 201–2)

Behind the mask

I needed to be able to manage myself extremely patiently in order to create the potential for knowledge to come to light. A murder had not actually occurred. However, the threat of Heather being killed by the particular form of her illness probably directed my countertransference experience more into the realms of there being a culprit and a victim (there was certainly a body!). Since both were residing in Heather herself, 'resistance' was inevitable.

Clinical example 8.1(c)

Heather gradually became more overtly accepting of my involvement and approach but her ambivalence persisted. My arrival for her sessions would be greeted with at least a momentary look of hostility, distaste or disgust (comparable with the assault on my own olfactory sense). Progress was facilitated by a slip of the tongue which I made.

One morning, Heather looked up as I entered her room, smiled but then looked momentarily shocked. I responded with a smile and said 'Yes it's me...a *face* worse than death'. Immediately I had said it, we both laughed, instantly recognising my mistake. My unconscious was far more astute than all my intellectualising capacities in understanding her fears. Something in the immediate visual impact of the object, the change from the having-not-been-there to the being-there was a 'fate worse than death': that was the problem. The idea of 'the fate/face worse than death' became part of our culture and language together.

This illustrates another core theme of psychosomatic problems, the inability to manage change. For Heather there was rarely ease in any transition. Unanticipated change virtually always disrupted her. There was seldom such a thing as a 'nice surprise' or 'a manageable shock'. The need to maintain internal control meant seeking to limit change through attempting to control the outside world. In consequence other people experience these patients as 'controlling'. But there is a fine line between judging that this is a last-ditch defence against disaster rather than a form of relating which gives pleasure in the control and even subjugation of someone else. It is particularly difficult to consider desperation rather than manipulation when it can be so unpleasant to be on the receiving end. This accounts, I believe, for much of the antipathy which arises from practitioners towards these patients. It can be easier to react against the patient as wilful rather than vulnerable.

Transitional mechanisms assist coping with change. The child who can 'drop off' to sleep without mother if she has her teddy bear has achieved some mastery: she can manage the transition from being 'an awake person' to being 'an asleep person' without a fear of loss of sense of continuity. But the component of obsessional disorders which is resistance to change has its roots in the same soil and at times there will be manifestations in MUS which are indistinguishable from this, at least in their surface manifestations.

Lord of the Rings

Having a conversation with Heather was not easy: for her to initiate a process was sometimes impossible or intolerable. I had to strike a careful balance between attempting to initiate conversations and maintaining a silence out of which something might become possible for her. What was required was the offer of a potential meeting place in words into which she might eventually be able to emerge safely – a rendezvous point.

Magagna (2000) found periods of silence to be an almost universal experience in work with eating disordered young people and described technical issues in psychoanalytic psychotherapy. Christie (2000), a cognitive behavioural therapist working with the same group of patients, states 'To impose ... control over the therapeutic experience may require them to be silent. Sitting with a child in silence for an hour feels extremely persecutory ... An inability to think in an abstract way may also make it hard for the child to think about her problems.'

It was never easy to judge whether or not my response to Heather's silence on any particular day or moment should be to remain silent or to attempt to initiate a conversation. The deadening quality meant that what I first needed to achieve was an internal conversation or even a thought, rather than aspiring to an interpersonal exchange.

The dramatic nature of her symptoms provided an easy point of contact particularly during those phases when the threat of death was present. However, this could itself become limiting or even boring – there are a limited number of permutations of enquiry and response to vomiting, blood sugars and electrolyte levels. The setting for therapy, Heather's room on the ward, was unusual and offered many opportunities for observation and comment. But how could I know what might be usefully capitalised upon for the therapeutic task rather than it being a stimulus to acting out in the countertransference?

Going by the book

Clinical example 8.1(d)

One day I noticed that Heather was reading *Lord of the Rings* (Tolkein 1954). I had read (and enjoyed) it many years earlier. I commented on it but without any reference to my enjoyment of it. The interchange about the book did not last long but the book became a reference point for us.

I took a position that for her to read it meant that she would have an experience of it and in that experience we might find meaning. This might give us a meeting point, which, in turn, might help in understanding her in her illness. Heather was very limited in what she could say about the story even in as far as describing the content let alone extending this into meaning.

This put me in the position of having to draw explicitly on my own memories of the book and gradually to introduce more of what I pieced together about its possible significance. This meant that I was taking the initiative in a way that would not usually feel correct in psychotherapy. However, it felt necessary if I was to be of use to Heather. *Lord of the Rings* became central to my thinking about Heather and the nature of the defence mechanisms involved in psychosomatic presentations in general. It offers a model of a mind at work in the service of the patient.

The ring defence: a double-edged sword

The central issue in *Lord of the Rings* is the unusual powers the ring bestows on its possessor. When worn on the finger, the ring makes the wearer invisible.[4] It has the potential to be a life-saving defence. It could also leave others who were in conflict with the wearer feeling threatened by not being able to see him: they then experienced the threat of knowing that they might now be prey not hunter.

However, using the ring is not without adverse effects. It exerts power over the owner both through simple ownership and through its use: this power could corrupt both the physical form and the moral integrity of the owner. Day (1994: 95, 154) described its effect on one of the central characters: 'Gollum [was] turned into a tormented ghoul ... enslaved [by its] power...' and '[it] seemed to possess Gollum more than Gollum possessed the ring...'. Tolkien (1954: 154) summarised Gollum's relationship with the ring: 'He hated it and loved it, as he hated and loved himself. He could not get rid of it. He had no will left in the matter.' Ultimately Gollum, corrupted physically and spiritually, died because of his desire to regain ownership of the ring.

The ring's properties are directly analogous to the defensive properties of Heather's physical symptoms, including the way in which they took on a life of their own. The symptoms served to make invisible, and provide a refuge for her It. Furthermore, they left the sense of danger (of causing harm) residing in others. Here was a reversal of experience, the turning of overwhelming vulnerability into potentially omnipotent threat: a *defensive, projective attack* on the object. It is this *unconscious attack* which is often misinterpreted as overt aggression and the accompanying lack of emotion and vitality even misinterpreted as *belle indifference.*

171

The perpetuation of the 'ring defence' is a corrupting force. It has a compelling, addictive quality if it gives power and control over others. These processes ruled Heather's life rather than being a means of living a fulfilling life. Possessing and using them can feed a perverse process, usually unconscious but sometimes conscious, i.e. there is an investment in (cathexis of) the defence. Any sense of uncertainty and unsafety is located elsewhere, in the object. For the subject, this provides the 'safe haven' of unconscious conflict management but it does not provide resolution. In addition, there is the potential for the secondary cathexis to lead to it 'taking on a life of its own'. These themes, couched within the culture and language for conversation which I developed with Heather (and her mother), became 'usable currency' in our work together.

Such defences do not let go readily. To attempt to 'remove' them threatens to bring about a return of the raw original state of powerlessness and torment which had had to be obliterated. Hence therapeutic endeavour is met with a ferocity accorded to the absolute enemy. The importance of making this explicit in the establishment of clinical contact with children and their parents and using it as a therapeutic tool is discussed below.

The heart of the matter

Clinical example 8.1(e)

Heather had been extremely ill when I had last seen her. Her heart rhythm was affected by severe electrolyte imbalance and she was experiencing ectopic beats. The nature of the imbalance meant that if this tipped over into a more dangerous arrhythmia it would not be possible to resuscitate her. She would die.

I felt it was important to her that I attended as usual. On entering the room, I saw Heather sitting by the window and on the window sill just above her head was a heart monitor. While looking at her face, I also looked at her heart rhythm observing any ectopic beats displayed on the screen.

Knowing what it was reasonable to do felt impossible. We sat quietly but I did make a few comments. These were relatively 'neutral' 'space-fillers' (or, perhaps, attempts at 'space-creators') which served as acknowledgements of our immediate presence together in the situation and our continuity of contact. However, the effect of even the simplest of comments was displayed above her head as an increased heart rate and increased numbers of ectopic beats. More or less any assertion of my self in her presence seemed manifestly to be a potential threat to her life. Never have I experienced Winnicott's description of the importance of 'being' as opposed to 'doing' more emphatically.

The experience of being with Heather and the cardiac monitor embodied the raw essence of her fragile hold on life in its fullest psychosomatic sense – sitting there with her, seeing the record of her heart beats, regular and ectopic, knowing and seeing that anything could affect them. She had no protection against sounds, not even sounds without apparent cognitive or emotional meaning. My actions and her continuing life were profoundly interconnected.

As a psychiatrist the closest one usually comes to potentially being decisive in matters of life and death is when trying to come between a suicidal patient's self-destructive thoughts, feelings and impulses and their ability to act on them. In the latter situation it is perhaps easier to have a sense of the patient as agent although even here problems ensue if there is not fuller reflection on notions of 'free will'.[5] In the psychosomatic constellation, what has to be held on to even more tenaciously is that the patient is in the power of something that cannot be grappled with in the ordinary language of 'agency' even though it is *of* the patient. The 'agent' is the 'It' which 'In accordance with its own infallible purpose ... creates speech, breathing, sleeping, work and joy and rest and love and grief, always with correct judgement, always purposefully, and always with full success, and finally, when he has lived long enough, it kills him' (Groddeck, quoted in Symington 1986: 149). Whereas previously I had possessed 'a *face* worse than death', I now possessed a voice which could be executioner – a terrifying expression of power and powerlessness intertwined.

I was never able properly to explore the transferential origins of Heather's illness. It was clear that her mother had been isolated and unsupported and in significant difficulties emotionally when Heather was an infant. As a toddler Heather had an episode of acute illness which it was feared could be life-threatening and there was a tormenting wait for the results of medical tests. In the pre-school period, Heather was described as having uncontainable temper tantrums and in her primary school she had had times when she was unable to separate from her mother. The threat of disruption to continuity of being and relating had clearly been a theme.

The meeting place is the hiding place

Symptoms are both the expression and the masking of elements of mental life. Symptoms are the place where the underlying psychopathology is manifest and where it is hidden. Similarly, 'Words both reveal and conceal thought and emotion' (Sharpe 1940: 155).

Vanessa and Heather illustrate the difficulty of feeling that one has truly been able to grasp the problem. With Vanessa, creating the diagnostic identity of 'Bert' was an attempt to bring to knowledge (into the light of day) the nature of Vanessa's illness. He represented the internally differentiated complex whose identity continued to be elusive but who made his presence felt. We usually found him in Vanessa's throat and ears, but he could be difficult to really pin down, i.e. 'know' him. He slipped away and re-emerged elsewhere. At certain times, he needed us to remember him, to keep him in mind, whilst he still attempted to live a life of his own, battling to exist in a world with the old, persecutory or persecuting but familiar rules. But he also needed us to know that we did not know him, and that he was in charge of that experience in us – an interminable process of hide-and-seek.

Ultimately, playing hide-and-seek is not *playful* if there is only not-finding or not-being-found: there is no mutuality, no mastery of the tension inherent in being lost or found. There can be no sense of achievement in the growing capacity to use abilities in either role. To be a game, it requires the period of being in the not-finding/not-being-found state to be sufficient to make this experience containable without unmanageable threat. The denouement, the experience of being a person who will be found and who can find, is essential. It allows an expression of ambivalence in the relationship. It expresses the feelings of wanting to be with and not wanting to be with someone. It is a mechanism which provides for both the potential excitement in the state of mastery of the other/mastery of the state of persecutory anxiety and for the satisfaction and potential pleasure of the state of coming-to-be-together.

Vanessa was able to move to a state where her experience was one of depression rather than only bodily states (see *Clinical example 7.1(g)*). In 're-finding' Bert in her relationship with me and simultaneously re-finding me through writing to me, she was able to 'find it in herself' to contend with this state. Although this was still not transformed into a *game* of hide-and-seek, it had become a process of lost-**and**-found.

Heather's symptoms never relented. There were some periods of relative freedom from symptoms but these were never maintained. However, she came to experience me as trustworthy despite this. Something about my striving to continue to be available to her physically and psychologically despite the nature of the experience was important. I think an essential ingredient in this was my appreciation of her being the victim of her illness rather than the agent of it. I was capable of taking a position of *negative culpability*. In such situations, to seek a single cause and apportion blame is futile and morally questionable.

Negative culpability allied with *negative capability*[6] produce a position of timely open-mindedness which allows data and information to be taken in without being acted upon precipitately. This reduces the likelihood of prematurely focusing attention, selecting some *raw* data and hastily excluding others. This combination is the foundation of good scientific method and *psychoanalytic neutrality*.

Alexythymia, athymylexia or aphorylexia?

Psychosomatic presentations cannot be described adequately by a focus on *feelings* and their relationship with words. The constituents are a failure:

- to hold inner *experiences* in the mind
- to capture experience in words in the inner world
- to put inner experiences in the interpersonal sphere
- to put experience into words in a form which can be understood by others
- for the subject to experience the communication as having been accurately enough received.

This formulation allows of a number of contributory factors with variable significance or impact. In certain areas of mental life there may have been a fundamental failure to develop the ability to hold things in mind. There may be states of mind during which this capacity is lost for a time because of internal factors, interpersonal factors or external events, or an admixture of these.

Underlying conflicts in relation to tolerating 'not-knowing' or 'not-being-known' in psychical states which were originally experienced as 'a fate worse than death' are fundamental components of MUS. My formulation is consistent with McDougall's (1989: 93–4) finding: 'I came to the conclusion that my patients, unable to repress the ideas linked to emotional pain and equally unable to project these feelings delusionally onto the representations of other people, simply ejected them from consciousness. They were not suffering from an inability to experience or express emotion, but from an inability to contain and reflect over an *excess* of affective experience.' The process is one of removal from (obliteration of) experience. A corollary of this is that we need to re-examine the use of the word *alexythymia* in order to highlight a crucial conceptual difference which needs to be considered.

The definition of alexithymia focuses on words and feelings. The prefix, *alex–* indicates 'no words'. The suffix *–thymia* generally connotes 'feelings' although it may also indicate something unpleasant, for example dysthymia. Webster's dictionary (1993) also gives the original Greek root as 'thymos ... spirit, mind, courage'. These do not approach sufficiently closely to the complex with which I am struggling nor, I believe, do they capture McDougall's proposition. A different word is needed.

Dysphoria describes a state of mental unease or discomfort. It is derived from the Greek *dysphoros* which in turn is derived from *pherein*, to bear. What needs to be captured is a state in which there are no words with which to communicate what the person is having to bear – *alexyphoria*. However, even this cannot capture fully the mechanisms that result in there being a state of absence of conscious experience to put into words: perhaps *aphorylexia* approximates more closely.

Siobhan (*Clinical example 7.2*) described *aphorylexia* very clearly: 'I have given you back the papers just as they were because **I feel blank!**' Siobhan was able to use words to communicate very powerfully about her feelings of unhappiness with her plight and her anger about the therapists not making her feel better: but in other areas of her mental life there was no mental experience, a blank. (Interestingly, when Siobhan was asked subsequently to think of a name for her illness, she decided upon 'Murder'.)

It may be folly to attempt to define a single word to describe this phenomenon since any word must ultimately reflect the *in*ability of language to get close to capturing what has to be borne in mind in trying to work with what cannot be borne in mind.

'Dual' or 'duel' diagnosis?

Remaining open to understanding patients involves thinking of the possibility of 'dual diagnosis'. A patient with a physically identifiable disorder may have an additional disorder. Ultimately the value of classificatory systems lies in their clinical usefulness. Sometimes systems may appear to be in opposition but if used as hypotheses and formulations to be compared and contrasted they may be complementary. They may orientate us through a process of triangulation. Triangulation in navigation can achieve a precise location but realistically it defines an area in which something or someone can be found. By analogy we can make allowance for the inherent inaccuracy of tools (mechanical and human) and of changes during the time it takes to make our observations by cross-referencing. This can be particularly useful in complex cases.

Clinical example 8.2(a)

Yasmin was 15 years old when she had abdominal symptoms. Investigation showed some abnormalities: she was then seen by a consultant paediatrician who referred her for psychiatric assessment. The paediatrician explained in the referral that generally she would have awaited the results of all the tests before initiation of treatment. The likely diagnosis was one which could produce a depressive picture because of its general debilitating effects. These symptoms usually remitted soon after treatment was instituted. However there was some quality in Yasmin's presentation, particularly the intensity of her low mood, which made her feel she should not delay. I saw Yasmin and understood why my paediatric colleague had made the referral as soon as possible.

The wait for a definitive diagnosis was protracted. This made it very complicated – this was a different situation. The expectation was of 'medically explained symptoms', the treatment of which was

---

highly likely to lead to alleviation of psychological symptoms. But as the wait extended we discussed whether some symptomatic treatment might be of benefit. The gastrointestinal specialist was reluctant to instigate specific treatment on the basis of a presumptive diagnosis in case the results were equivocal and further tests were needed. I offered some medication to help her sleep – this was acceptable to her and her mother. A trial of antidepressants was started even though the depressive features were expected to be a secondary effect rather than this being a situation of 'dual diagnosis'.

Consultations with Yasmin and her mother (*Clinical example 10.5*) presented many of the psychodynamic issues with which I was familiar from the work with children and adolescents with MUS. I had also found that similar dynamic issues arose with girls with eating disorders. Yasmin demonstrated difficulties initiating processes; she needed her mother as both an advocate and the recipient of projections of uselessness and incompetence. There were some differences including the extent of overt expressions of active opposition rather than inaction or passive resistance.

Clinical example 8.2(b)

We were still awaiting completion of paediatric tests, after some had been abnormal but not characteristic of any disease. Yasmin's general behaviour was becoming more difficult. She was becoming secretive and rebellious at home and some of her activities became more worrying.

Although now displaying more frustration with me, she did also seem actively engaged, valuing my involvement. She was an intelligent girl so I thought it might be useful to articulate more of the diagnostic process dilemmas I had identified. I specifically explained my puzzlement that there were some processes occurring which I was used to seeing when there was no expectation of discovering any physical abnormality. I expanded on this by explaining how that experience was guiding me in the ways I was responding to Yasmin, her mother and other family members if they attended: my responses seemed to fit for them in terms of their predicament. I said that the patterns were similar when teenagers had specific difficulties with food and eating. Yasmin stated emphatically that she did not have anorexia.

I suggested that we could try some of the things I used in those other situations including seeking a name that Yasmin would feel was suitable as an interim diagnosis and writing down something about her symptoms – showing me what she had written if she wanted to.

Yasmin had taken to the idea that something was happening inside her that had taken on 'a life of its own': she decided that would be a suitable diagnostic label. She wrote the following and gave it to me to read at a subsequent consultation.

Clinical example 8.2(c)

'The thing inside me has a mind and life of its own. The only thing he doesn't have is his own body. So he takes over other peoples, and makes them suffer horribly. Thats his life. He enjoys it. While he has fun, I hurt more and more inside. Over time it becomes daily, and becomes a part of your life, like he's become a part of mine. He's taken over my life and my body. I can't control anything any more. I can't even control how I feel. I've grown to hate myself. Because of him, not by choice. He drains me, not in one, but in many ways. He takes away my meaning for life, so all I want is to be dead. He makes me think there is nothing to live for. He punishes me if I do something he doesn't like. I had to stay strong so people around me wouldn't worry about me. But the monster inside me is growing everyday and he weakens me. He hurts in several ways. Slowly ... I was dying a slow painful, delayed death ... I could feel it. One thing he absolutely loved was seeing me suffer. I had to be strong so no-one would realise I had to cover up my feeling and fears. I was alone. I had to fight him by myself. But that was all in the past. Things have started to change. Get better. He stops hurting me so much. He's dying himself. I'm hoping it'll be over soon ... then he strikes again. I'm scared. I'm hoping it's just a one off ... it is, until he strikes again the next day. The thing I wished wouldn't happen, my worse fear ... is as before. I'm right at the beginning of a never-ending story ... though the best thing is he's come back a lot weaker, which I'm hoping is a good sign...'

Yasmin's mother was worried about her unreliable eating patterns as well as her general behaviour which fitted with descriptions she knew of teenage girls with eating disorders. She confronted Yasmin. Yasmin vehemently denied any problem with food.

Clinical example 8.2(d)

Sometime later Yasmin's mother found some diaries in which Yasmin detailed her ways of restricting food intake along with other details consistent with anorexia nervosa. Yasmin then admitted to having problems which she did think were indicative of an eating disorder.

In the consultation when this came to light and in some subsequent appointments I described how I still did not understand why she had not been able to tell me. I juxtaposed the fact of what appeared to be her very active involvement with me as somebody useful and trustworthy with the fact that she had lied to me. I did not demand an answer nor take a 'moral stance' to her telling me untruths. Yasmin did not give an answer – I thought she did not have an answer to give.

Yasmin displayed many of the dynamic issues and surface symptoms of anorexia nervosa and of medically unexplained symptoms. The emphasis shifted at different times much as Vanessa's 'Bert' could move around. The rapidity of shift perhaps suggested a more general upheaval in Yasmin's development. It was not possible during the time of my involvement to ascertain whether this was likely to be a developmental crisis, perhaps precipitated or shaped by the gastrointestinal disease or a more profound developmental breakdown.

In retrospect, my diagnosis might have been 'Duel', to capture the battle between developmental progression and regression.

Through countertransference to therapeutic case management

The very nature of the psychosomatic disorders with which we come in contact can undermine the ability to experience and think. The essence of the underlying defence in the patient is to prevent experiencing and thinking because they are intolerable. It comes into play producing encapsulated areas of 'not-being', physical symptoms which interfere with everyday functioning but without transformation of this into death. Understanding this as a *psychological hibernation* captures the process of psychosomatic shut-down in the context of an environment which cannot provide for more active living and in which the environmental characteristics themselves represent a danger. A state of hibernation is one from which *living*, as defined by existing and developing as an individual who can experience their inner and outer worlds with sufficient sense of agency, tolerability and potential satisfaction, can still re-emerge from *life* as a 'pure' physiological process. The first task for the clinician is to manage the impact of the psychosomatic complex upon him or herself, avoiding the extremes of hibernation or inappropriate activity. Then the countertransference processes can be translated to provide a matrix of containment and holistic therapeutic management in which living can re-emerge in that life.

Working with professional colleagues

Psychoanalytic psychotherapy places the therapist into the full glare, shadow and/or focus of the patient's transferences and projections. Unconscious phenomena do not only impact upon professionals in the psychotherapy room. They are present in everyday life and are manifest in a variety of ways in any relationships that have particular import. This applies not only to intimate affectional relationships, but also in contacts with health professionals where the intimacy of the body and its functions, and the sense that there is something wrong, are the currency of interchange. These relationships do not undergo the same crystallisations and transformations which occur in psychotherapy or psychiatric relationships. Nevertheless patient care can be enhanced by attunements and adaptations which are informed by the extended understanding derived from appreciation of these unconscious processes. 'Psychoanalytically informed therapeutic case management' is the briefest term I have so far been able to formulate for this.

Developing the ability to contend with states of 'not-knowing' is an essential aspect of the human condition. Groddeck described this process of change from 'overestimat[ing] consciousness and reason' as 'the loss of illusions' (1925: 153). If paediatric staff were held in the full grasp of the countertransference of 'psychological hibernation', wards and clinics would be littered with sleeping doctors and nurses. This is not a common sight. However, other manifestations of its impact do still occur. Unhelpful activity in the form of medical tests or procedures may occur: omnipotent attributions of causation may be formulated. A regular experience is to hear of a new professional involvement and an idealised investment in 'the specialist' who is deemed to know exactly what the problem is and exactly what to do. A new professional may express a very clear and precise diagnostic formulation without the presence of doubt or room for debate, perhaps even puzzlement over why something so obvious was not recognised before (the everyday phrase 'it goes without saying!' encapsulates this position and also links to the underlying dynamic that words do not operate very effectively in this arena). The paediatric team is therefore as much in need of the tools to handle states of not-knowing as the mental health specialist.

As mental health specialists working alongside our colleagues from other specialities we have to delineate what each of us does and does not know in order to establish who is likely to be most use at various points. The interprofessional task is to manage this in order then to identify in which arenas 'therapeutic activity' is required, the physical or the psychological, and who therefore should be taking the lead role at which points. We need our paediatric colleagues to be able to identify and explain:

- that all necessary attention has been paid to the history, physical examination and investigation

- in order that a reasonable professional opinion can be given that there is no evidence of a physically definable illness which represents a danger to the patient
- that there is no evidence that further physical investigation should be carried out
- and that, even though the physician cannot give an explanation of why the child has these symptoms, she can confidently recommend the involvement of a mental health specialist.

The paediatrician should be confident enough to say, 'Although I cannot explain exactly why you have/your child has these particular symptoms, I do feel confident that there are no indicators that further tests should be done and there is no evidence of a dangerous physical cause for the illness. In these situations I need the help of the mental health specialist.'

Subsequently, we need the continued availability of the paediatrician. We may find ourselves wondering if a change of symptoms needs re-appraisal by the paediatrician. We may feel that the only mechanism for communication is the 'laying on of hands' by the paediatrician in order to demonstrate the fact that the body is being held in mind, i.e. the *primary (sensory) process route* may still be needed.

What can be particularly difficult to demonstrate explicitly is that the process of *containment* is an active internal state since it may appear to be a state of inactivity. This requires the development of a particular form of relationship between those whose expertise lies in the arena of the physical and those whose expertise is in the realm of the mental. The translation of this into the shared area of practice lies in the explicit use of this understanding with each other and with the patient and parent. 'Referral to the psychiatrist' needs to be translated as 'request for involvement of the psychiatrist' in order to capture the need for the involvement of specialists from both arenas. In a similar vein, I will always explain to the paediatrician and to the patient and their parents that I need the continuing availability of the paediatrician. The purpose of this is to address the omnipotent mechanisms at the heart of the presentation. All clinicians need to model that they can explore and define the boundaries of their ability without equating this with impotence. As McGinn (1999: 76) states, 'knowledge of one's constitutional limitations is often valuable and useful knowledge, leading either to calm resignation or to a better strategy for overcoming a problem. Sticking your head in the sand and insisting on your cognitive perfection is hardly the sensible response to a palpable intellectual shortcoming. A clear-sighted admission of ignorance is never a bad thing.'

Working with children and parents

Symptoms may make fundamental inroads into all areas of the life of the child and other family members. The child is contending with the symptoms and the demands of the environment in relation to these as well as developmental demands: for parents the experience is of seeing their child suffering or disabled in some way and feeling powerless to do anything about it despite their best efforts. Parents may find themselves in conflict about whether to challenge the child by forcing activities or to allow her to desist from them. The internal struggle of the child can manifest in conflict between the adults or in parental conflict with the child. Alternatively, conflict between parent and child may be avoided because there is a coming together through finding an external figure whom they believe has all the answers or in opposition to someone who is not of the same mind.

Clinicians have to face similar dilemmas and pressures as parents. Simultaneously there is a communication that there is something wrong which they have a responsibility to respond to and the feeling that whatever they do may be wrong (and therefore dangerous). The task is therefore complex, presenting inevitable and recurrent contradictions. The symptoms are the 'best solution' to psychic conflict that has emerged to that point; any change represents a threat so any response outside of expectations is a threat. This has to be addressed proactively.

It is essential that the child and parents are given the opportunity to tell the story of the illness without challenge. The way clinicians have been involved *prior to* the onset of current symptoms and *during* the current illness is an essential part of the emerging structure of the presentation. The possibility of successful engagement with the child and parents will have been affected already by the mode of operation of those professionals. Splitting may be manifest in the idealisation or denigration of individuals or their particular lines of approach. By explicitly presenting oneself in line with the formulation of 'knowing and not-knowing', it is possible to counteract some of these. I respond to recognisable patterns by describing those which I have come across before whilst acknowledging that every individual is different: I am therefore in familiar terrain even though the territory is fresh (see Chapter 4). I describe the key features I can recognise and the sense I have of what is likely to be present in conjunction with these, but state that I still need to look carefully at their personal situation and come to understand them better.

The paradox between the hope that I will provide a solution and the threat contained in challenging the symptoms needs to be made explicit. I build into my initial and continuing contacts with these young people and their families the statement 'If you do decide to use me, there will be times when it feels like **I'm** the problem.' This was a change from the form I had previously used – 'If you do decide to use me, there will be times when *you* will feel like *I* am the problem.' Put in the former terms it is an explicit statement to the patient and their parents about my clinical knowledge and experience. It is also an implicit reminder to me that this is going to be a countertransference experience, i.e. I will have to struggle with the feeling that I *am* the problem: an enemy working in some way towards the downfall of her/him/them. I also specifically cite the issues formulated with the paediatricians, emphasising the suffering and the intrusion into life which the symptoms make alongside the idea of 'safely not-knowing'. I describe my role as being a 'specialist in not-knowing'.

The primary task then becomes one of attempting *translation* as opposed to *interpretation*. There are two principal tools in this, metaphor and a process of reflection and articulation of how one is striving to understand. The aim is to demonstrate acceptance and confirmation of the experience of the individual without this being presented as meaning agreement with their underlying beliefs whether these are considered pathological or healthy.

Using metaphor

The clinical process is one of searching for those responses which may 'capture' sufficient experience of the patient or parent, or both, in order that there is a potential 'meeting of minds'. In line with the pattern of inherent simultaneous or recurrent disqualification, this has to be couched in terms which represent the least threat to integrity and relatedness or the sense of being a person with a mind and body of one's own. The choice of metaphor may be from everyday usage or there may be a process of construction between patient, parent and professional. The expansion of the metaphor to look at its literal meaning illuminates the underlying psychic experience being defended against. Two which are commonly useful illustrate this.

Walking a tightrope: The delicate balancing act calls upon physical and mental discipline and strength in the face of the threat of serious damage if they stop operating. There is minimal margin for error, although a slip may be recovered from (e.g. by grabbing hold of the rope). However, recovering the former equilibrium, albeit unstable, does not appear likely.

On a knife-edge: This encapsulates some of the same issues as the tightrope but here the actual place where one 'finds one's feet' could also be dangerous rather than a refuge. To stand on this knife-edge is tantamount to denying the real purpose of a knife. A loss of balance leading to a fall to the side is comparable to the fall from the tightrope. A fall forwards or backwards brings the threat of being cut by the knife, possibly sliced in two; trying to grab the knife blade to prevent the fall brings the same threat to bodily integrity without any likelihood of being able to hold on.

These capture the lack of sense of a safe, firm foundation, the threat of imminent catastrophe and need for a focus on achieving physical safety. They truly recognise the gravity of the situation.

Having a mind of one's own

Development is reliant on being able to identify similarities and differences. For some people, recognition of difference can be a source of pleasure in itself and they make seek novelty, perhaps even as end in itself. However, for others the new or unexpected, and therefore different and unknown, may contain only threat.

As demonstrated by Heather's material, the possibility of something being a *pleasant* surprise may not exist. Instead, 'tightrope', 'knife-edge' or 'fate/face worse than death' experiences govern. For such people, any change or difference can initiate the defence mechanisms described. Change can be from the familiar to the unfamiliar or even the change from the familiar to the familiar when the difficulty resides more in managing the actual process of change rather than the content of either setting. This is why so many of the children with MUS are described as 'school avoidant' even though there may not be specifically identifiable stressors in either setting. What may not be manageable is the change between these most usual of environments. For some the lack of a sense of a trustworthy place to be in *next* means that going to sleep may be difficult: getting out of bed can be a mountain to climb because changing from being an 'in-bed person' to an 'out-of-bed person' feels insuperable. Although encopresis has been addressed separately in the previous chapter, it is a form of MUS. A recurrent scenario is of school staff insisting the child must be soiling at home, with parents denying this on the basis that the child arrives home having soiled and must therefore have soiled at school. Both sides need to appreciate that the child has been in a third place – neither in school nor at home. In being in transition, they have been a 'not-at-home-and-not-at-school person'. There may be external threat to the child on his journey but it may be that 'simple' change and transition is the problem. Adults need to understand this and avoid inadvertently enacting 'out of sight, out of mind'.

Difference also involves experiencing self and other as truly separate. When a parent seems to do all the talking, how do we to know if we are obtaining a proper report of symptoms? Is the parent speaking for the child or for herself? Or are they both 'of one mind'? Seeking people who are 'of a like mind', for example, in relation to their beliefs about the cause of the illness, can be a powerful defence mechanism. The sense of 'being known' can give temporary relief as it can consolidate assumptions of being understood without relying on verbal communication. Relationships can be built on the basis of 'it goes without saying'. 'Alexythymia', 'alexyphoria' or 'aphorylexia' can be bypassed. However, finding these relationships may serve to perpetuate symptoms through fixing them in time. Such a process can be a powerful method for embedding and feeding symptoms.

The synthesis of these elements brings about an approach which strives to create a space in which feelings consequent upon change and difference linked with bodily states can be lived with, even if they are not understood. Being acknowledged as a separate person is acknowledging difference. The threat inherent in separation-individuation must be managed without resorting to denial of difference or attempting to seduce or bully the person into the same way of thinking. Even agreement contains its own complexity since it may be confused with 'being of the same mind' rather than there being two or more minds with the same beliefs. This process of striving to understand whilst acknowledging that we cannot be the 'same as' needs to be made explicit in the clinical setting.

These complicated dynamics can be translated into ordinary language. In conjunction with the presentation of one's understanding to child and parents, the question 'Does it sound like *you* I am talking about ... or at least a bit like you?' carries the sense of a process of 'coming to know better' rather than absolute states of 'being known or not-known'.

The essence is that we can only ever achieve good-enough understanding. In Groddeck's (1925: 201) words: 'all this and more needs to be taken into account if one wants to get the meaning of this illness approximately right'.

Conclusions

From a psychodynamic perspective the conceptualisation of medically unexplained symptoms in children and adolescents can be expanded to include those problems relating to bodily functions of 'intake or out-put', for example eating disorders, defecation problems. The apparent wilfulness of opposition or resistance is either a direct defence against internal 'out-of-controlness' or the consequence of an internal process taking on a momentum (a life) of its own. Even where there does seem to be 'secondary gain' this still constitutes a process which takes on a life of its own: the difference is the youngster may not feel conflicted about it.

In listening to patients and parents or to others who are working with them I have come to recognise 'familiar terrain'. Patterns unfold in a way which feels familiar or they may throw light on something new. Yet, what is also always re-emphasised is the crucial importance of learning how to handle what is not known. The crucial question is 'How can I be confident that the sense of familiarity, of "knowingness", is not a manifestation of the engendering of omnipotent mechanisms rather than truly a reflection of having learnt from experience?'

Simultaneously maintaining a reflective stance and managing uncertainty is difficult. There is a danger of becoming tied up in knots by an obsessional doing and undoing or a circular 'disqualification by consideration' as an enactment of the countertransference. Intellectual scrutiny and investigation become stifled. For the patient and parent this manifests in the way in which dread turns every communication (whether internal or interpersonal) into its own disqualification. It can feel like 'Damned if I do, damned if I don't!'

Managing these complex dynamics is essential for professional integrity, for one's patients' benefit and in supporting parents in their care of their children. It is through this that patients can experience good-enough containment and internalise it with consequent enhanced access to their own developmental potential. What was once a threat to the primitive ego structure, reliant on its own omnipotent mechanisms whilst actually protected by external care, can become a pleasure. In 'finding it in oneself' to have the capability to meet and know different experiences in life there can be simple pleasure and developmental gain. The 'fate/face worse than death' can be transformed into a novel source of interest and enjoyment, because mastery of the internal turbulence or threat can be experienced in safety.

As mental health specialists, we must appreciate the experiential threat we represent by being containers for danger. We need to identify familiar terrain but recognise what is new territory and needs mapping. To continue the analogy, we are not trying to invade anyone's territory. By accompanying children, parents and colleagues, we contribute by tolerating the unknown. If we can avoid being ruled by our own or other people's phantasies of omniscience or omnipotence realistic progress can be made.

We need the continued availability and active involvement of paediatricians and other child health practitioners for the times when the quality of 'not-knowing' changes. The concreteness of their laying on of hands may be needed to evaluate if the symptoms have any possible significance in their specialist sphere. This makes it less likely that we will engage in unhelpful or even dangerous activity or premature rejection of cases where no apparently complete psychiatric or psychodynamic formulation presents itself.

A central task of the mental health specialist is to contend with the pressures, whether conscious and unconscious, to resort to modes of operating which automatically equate uncertainty with uselessness and danger. In order to be of use to the patient, we must become specialists not only in the knowledge-base of child and adolescent psychopathology, but also in 'not-knowing'.

9

UNTRANQUILITIS

Cathy was 13 years old when I first met her and 18 when I said 'goodbye'. This chapter is first and foremost hers. She prepared detailed accounts of what she wanted me and other people to know about her experience. Her hope is that it will help other people. (Some of the original material could not be produced very clearly for technical reasons but it is included to convey how Cathy wanted to communicate about her experience.)

I was asked to see Cathy for a second opinion when her medically unexplained symptoms persisted and became extremely disabling. She was generally quietly spoken although occasionally raised her voice. Often she did not say much. Sometimes she appeared reluctant about attending and at other times relieved by my persistent involvement. Usually if I brought up something new Cathy responded with some reservation but she was able to consider the idea of providing the name for her diagnosis. She took me by surprise when she arrived next time with both a name for her illness and an acrostic.

Other symptoms

fevers (hot and cold): hands and feet are always cold; twitching, mostly of feet: muscles feel tired; memory loss: loss of concentration; loss of appetite; headaches; lack of energy; abdominal pain; dizziness (inside and outside)

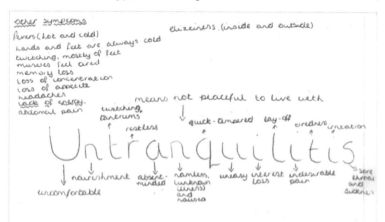

Figure 13

U – uncomfortable
N – nourishment
T – twitching + tantrums
R – restless
A – absent-minded
N – nameless (unknown illness) and nausea
Q – quick tempered
U – uneasy
I – interest loss
L – lay-off
I – indesirable pain
T – tiredness
I – irritation
S – sore throat and sickness

Cathy could rarely initiate conversations and gave little elaboration. She could however respond to enquiries about her interests. She had a fascination with horror movies and became much more animated on this topic than on others. I told her that if she would like to write something down about this, I'd be interested to read what she wrote if she wanted me to.

She wrote:

To Dr Sutton,
I like horror movies because they play with your mind and they keep your mind racing thinking who's the killer? Who's going to be killed next? Because they hook you and keep my mind off my symptoms sometimes.

When I've watched the film I feel inspired (not to kill!) but to try different things in life, like in The Haunting she decides to take up an insomnia course because she can't sleep so she stays at a big mansion with the other members and they try to help her so these films are very inspiring. I shouldn't stick to routine so much! Do something I've never done before – just like she did.
Cathy

I replied:

Dear Cathy
What an interesting letter. Not very long but with so much in it!

I think the idea that something plays with your mind is important. Horror films can be scary but you can hang on to the fact that they are not true – you can always know you'll be safe even if sometimes in the middle of the film you might forget it for a moment. I think there is something a bit the same about 'Untranquilitis' – it gives you 'horror' feelings but in your body so it's difficult to think that there could be anywhere that really is safe and where you can feel you've got it in you to get through the horrors to feel safe and strong all at the same time.

I wonder what a film called 'Untranquilitis' would be like! Could 'Untranquilitis' be a name, perhaps a secret name a character has for himself or herself? What about trying a story-line – think who the characters in the film could be? If you tried it, it would certainly be a change of routine! One of the things about changing routines is that you might get taken by surprise. Now, if you keep things the same, you can at least try and stop them getting even worse. The problem is it might stop them getting even better! The BIG question is 'Do you believe there can be anything like a nice surprise?'

Best wishes

Dr Sutton

Cathy was something of an enigma for her school. Her attendance was very poor. She was behind academically but school felt this could be accounted for by lack of attendance. They thought she was academically talented although they did wonder about her social relating: her Year Head did ask if I thought she was autistic. Cathy described having difficulties following lessons and finding her way around school. In conjunction with this and experiences of children with MUS having unrecognised learning difficulties, I asked school to involve an educational psychologist. Her teachers were resistant to this so I arranged for psychometric testing by an experienced clinical psychologist. The results confirmed that she had a complex, uneven test profile. Her verbal score was 81 and her performance score 63 with an overall intelligence quotient in the low 70s. The pattern was consistent with the problems Cathy described. However, school remained reluctant to accept the formulation. Eventually I did persuade the education department of her need for special provision rather than obstinately insisting 'social inclusion' would be of benefit.[1]

Cathy lived a very different life from other teenagers. Her symptoms fluctuated and occasionally new ones emerged. One of the most alarming for her parents was that she began to cut her wrists: the cuts were not dangerous but they were numerous and disturbing to observe.

Cathy's ability to use her abilities was not robust even within the ordinary complexity of relationships, for example in the school setting. Away from that complexity she could produce the profound and articulate exposition in her acrostic and wanted to share it in the therapeutic relationship. The onset of wrist-cutting indicated that developmental pressures were causing internal turbulence and disequilibrium. The fact that the consequence was an attack on her body contained a paradox. Although not desirable in itself, wrist-cutting did present a picture in which a growing sense of agency in the face of adversity could be identified in Cathy. She was victim and perpetrator of an act rather than simply being at the mercy of 'Untranquilitis'. The lack of robustness in her ego-functioning, allied with the particular developmental profile, including her intellectual abilities profile, meant that she remained an enigma for all of us. Her functioning continued to take us by surprise.

One day Cathy presented me with a book she had written to explain her illness. Some of this was an update on 'Untranquilitis' but it also introduced a new diagnosis – 'Tranquilitis'. It is presented here in its entirety.

Untranquilitis

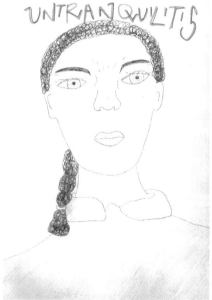 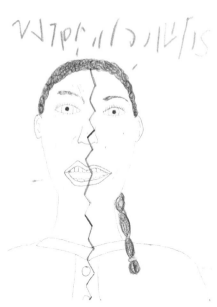

Figure 14   *Figure 15*

This folder contains:
*UNTRANQUILITIS – THE
STORY
* UNTRANQUILITIS – WHAT
IS IT?
* UNTRANQUILITIS –
THOUGHTS + FEELINGS +
MORE

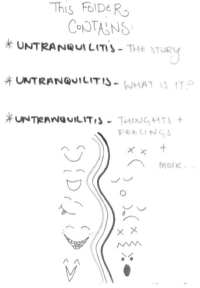

Figure 16

INTRODUCTION

I hope the story of Untranquilitis gives a clearer understanding on how I cope with this illness and the problems I have to face each day. 'Untranquilitis – what is it?' explains what I think Untranquilitis is and the symptoms of it and how the word 'Untranquilitis' fits perfectly with this illness and why I chose it. 'Untranquilitis – thoughts and feelings' explains how having tranquilitis makes me feel and the emotions that I feel mostly every day. I hope writing these things will be the key to finding out what untranquilitis really is and even how to cure it.

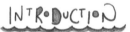

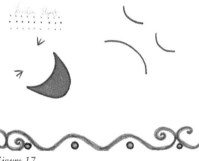

Figure 17

UNTRANQUILITIS

The story gives a clearer understanding on how I cope with my illness each day or if I don't know how to cope what do I do, how do I handle school and my symptoms? What about friends? Do I talk to them about my illness, do they know how bad it is for me? Do they notice my constant switches? Well it's all here in my story. A day in the life of me: can you handle it? Maybe not. Enjoy.

Please turn over

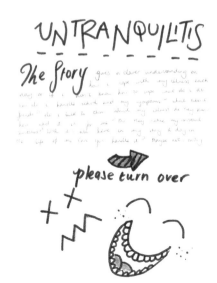

Figure 18

Transcript of subsequent pages

'Sorry what did you say?' I turned to Mum. She had a small basket of dirty clothes in her hands. She pointed to some cups that were on the window sill.

'Move those cups. Tidy this room and Cathy. Cathy?'

'Yes Mum' I said.

'What are you doing?' She said, staring down at the sheets of paper I had in front of me.

'Work.' I said. Then I paused 'What did you say before?'

'Just tidy your room.' She sighed and walked out the room.

Fifteen minutes later she came back up and the cups were still there. She carried them downstairs tutting and mumbling some words. I stared down at my work. I had done two pages. Why should I have to do this work? I thought, I think this was the untranquilitis thinking! Another part of me started thinking why don't I just get this finished: more work means more time for other things. Gosh it's just like having the Devil and the angel!

When I had finished my work I went downstairs and asked if I could read the newspaper. Mum said no and you practically hear my blood boiling! 'Why?!' I said 'Why can't I? I've done my work.' I said increasing my tone. I kept on pestering her until she gave me an answer.

'Are you in school? Well then you can't read the newspaper,' she said in a soft tone, which irritated me even more.

I slammed the kitchen door, slammed the living-room door shut too then I stamped up the stairs one by one. Screamed, and slammed my door a couple of times then I started crying, angry tears. When I cry I'm angry most of the time, I don't even feel upset but I don't know where these sudden bursts of anger come from. Mum said I had to release my anger in another way. But that's what I did when I was cutting my arms but now I can't do that I get frustrated and angry with the tiniest things.

Afterwards I went back downstairs and said sorry. But I was always saying sorry, I didn't know how to control my own temper. I went upstairs and started to read a book, Woman Killers, it was really good. I couldn't believe some of the reasons they would kill people for. I wouldn't ever hurt somebody like that, only if it was in self defence but some of them were mental and very bizarre. I closed the book and lied down on my bed, my head was thumping. I rubbed where the pain was but it still remained.

It was Saturday and I was on the Sims. It was great controlling little virtual people. My brother bounced into the room singing a song.

'Cathy. Can I have a go?' he said.

'Yes. One minute Jason.' I said focusing harder on the computer screen.

'The Grim Reeper came on my family because there was a massive fire' he said not pronouncing massive properly.

'We're going to the shopping mall' he said leaning on the back of my chair.

'We are?' I said. How did I feel? I had a bit of a stomach ache. Erm … yes I'll go. I need to get out. It'll make everyone a bit more calmer anyway. I get in the car not making and keep my mouth shut most of the way there but I'll occasionally ask questions about the latest pop bands, films and books. On the way I start panicking a bit but I take a few deep breaths and now I'm here.

'Can I go to the model shop?' Jason asks pulling Dad's sleeve.

'Maybe' he says.

'I've read all them' I said pushing back some horror books. So we go to look at some scary DVDs. I pick up Child's Play and Jeepers Creepers 2 and then House of Wax. Mum rolls her eyes.

'Why don't you get a nice film?' she asks.

'Boring' I say picking up another DVD. 'I'll have this one' I say walking towards the queue. Oh I hate ques. I stand in the que it has a bar going round the edges so I feel quite trapped. I won't be able to go out of the que now I thought I'm sandwiched between two people. I start getting panicky again but I manage to get to the front of the que and pay for my DVD.

'Do you want a bag?' the woman asked. Her hair was really messy and her nose was bent, she seriously needed a nose job. 'Erm yes please.' I say and pay her the money. I'd done it!

It was Tuesday, I had science. The teacher kept on announcing that we had a seating plan and that we had to hang our coats and bags at the back. I was sitting next to Sandy. Of course I wasn't supposed to be but I was just waiting she would notice.

'Maybe I should go Sandy, she'll notice me anyway' I said grabbing my coat and bag.

'Ciya then' she said.

'Ciya.' I sat in my right seat and said hello to Shahida and clutched my bag and coat and put them under the table so the teacher couldn't see them. I felt a bit worried as I was now at the back and the door was right at the front.

'Where have you been then. I haven't seen you for ages' Shahida said. I thinked up an excuse and changed the subject quickly. 'I've taped some new songs on my phone,' I said. The teacher started the register.

'You did, have you got 50 per cent, outta control?'

'Yeah.'

'Cathy?' the teacher said.

'Yes miss' I said.

When she finished she came over to some girls and asked them to move their coats then she came over to me.

'Cathy, move your coat' she said.

I hesitated but moved it. I didn't want an argument, my head was throbbing. What would I do now if I needed to leave the classroom? I took a deep breath and focused on the science work in front of me, it looked like Japanese to me.

After class I hurried down one corridor and went in the canteen for my dinner but when I got there and saw all the people I felt dizzy and sick. I walked straight out. Where should I go? I went to the Head of Year's room but she wasn't in so I went past the unit and went to reception. There was no women at reception so I just signed my name in the book made sure no one was looking and quickly walked out of school. I just had to get out of school. I felt tense. I was breathing so hard and my heart was beating so hard against my chest that I thought it was going to fall out. I walked quickly and didn't look back at the school. I wondered if my parents were going to be at home so I texted them to tell them I was coming home. I waited at the bus stop but the bus didn't come so I walked all the way home. My head pounded as I walked up the path to my house. I heard the hoover and I felt really disappointed as I knocked at the door.

'What are you doing home?' Dad asked. I sighed. I was used to this but I couldn't explain why I had come home because I really didn't know mself. I just felt I had to and I'd felt really panicky. I came and sat down on the couch and rubbed my head. 'Whatever' I sighed.

It was three o'clock, Jason would be home soon.

'Mum can I have the Sims back?' I asked her.

'No!' she said.

'Please!'

'I said No!'

I ran upstairs and started crying, the tears flooded from my eyes a mixture of emotions, frustration, anger and sadness. Ten minutes later Jason raced up the stairs and asked if he could go on the Sims. My mind said no but I forced a yes.

The next day we went to Dr Suton's I tapped my fingers and hummed a song the way there. We arrived I got out and pressed the buzzer. It buzzed and we walked in. A pale woman asked who we were coming to see and Mum replied, she told us to sit in the waiting room. Then we saw Dr Suton, he gestured us upstairs. We sat down in our usual seats.

'How's things been lately?' he said looking at me. I burst out laughing for no reason.

'What's funny? Don't you understand what I was saying?' he said leaning back in his chair. I pulled the sleeves up and saw the cuts on my arms they were just scars now.

'Nothing' I said.

Mum started talking, she was saying how hard things had been lately. She looked a bit calmer today though usually she'd look really tense, her face was usually pink and she'd always fiddle with her hands. Dad was the same as he always is, chilled out, smiling, he looked like a Cheshire cat. I start laughing again.

'What has happened lately, Cathy?' Dr Sutton asked.

'erm… erm well things have been harder lately I suppose but it's the holidays now so I'm not really bothered'.

I looked at the clock it was nearly over, when I looked at Mum she started saying how ill she was getting with all the stress and worry from everything. I felt angry at that point. Why should I worry about her after what she's done? She didn't believe me when I told her I was ill, she said she got sick of me complaining Duh! I had an ILLNESS! My fingers tensed and I breathed the anger out of me but of course it was still there, at the pit of my stomach. I remember when Jason used to see me get upset and he'd think I was putting everyone did. Even the thick doctors I would love to throttle them it's so lucky they catched it when it was just going. Ha! Just going and they could have helped me way before that! I won't forgive anyone for this because this is why it's so hard for me to deal with it now because I'm so scared that I'll get it again and that no-one will believe. I take a lot of paracetamol too so I keep illnesses at bay but lately I've been cutting down on them.

It was the start of the holidays, I was in my room watching Child's Play 2. I felt sick and had a headache. Sometimes I would pray to god to make my symptoms go away, at my worst point I even wanted to commit suicide but if I did that I would be a coward and I'm not because I'm a fighter and if I so want people to understand then I need to write storys, do things and tell people how my life is so more people know what's it like to live with untranquilitis.

Did you understand

Untranquilitis?

If your still a bit puzzled

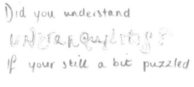

Read on...

U - unable to go out
N - no concentration
T - tired all the time
R - really bad headaches
A - abdominal pains
N - no energy
Q - queasy most of the time
U - unable to remember certain things
I - interaction difficulties
L - loss of sleep
I - ill most of the time
T - terrible migraines
I - interest loss
S - switching off

Figure 19

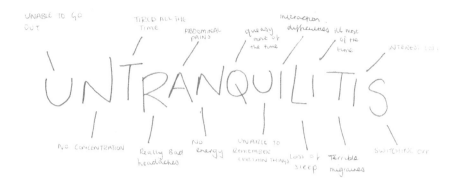

What is it?

Figure 20

UNTRANQUILITIS

Thoughts and feelings

Since I've had untranquilitis I've been on an emotional rollercoaster. Some days I will feel happy that I've gone to school. I've seen my friends or that I have gone out somewhere but on other days I can feel upset or down mainly because I have felt that the untranquilitis has beat me and if I feel really upset I cut my arms and start getting snappy with people and I release my anger out on them. Which will make them angry with me and we'll all start back at square one and think if we help each other then we can beat this untranquilitis once and for all then I will be able to help other people with the same thing.

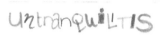

Figure 21

197

DO NOT HIDE YOURSELF AWAY,
SPEAK OUT
YOU ARE NOT ALONE.

UNTRANQUILITIS – what is it?
I think of untranquilitis as a part of me now, the other half.... It's like an unknown creature is trying to control my body and plague me with symptoms (headaches, stomach pains, dizziness etc). Another symptom after another can be frustrating, this is one of the reasons why I started to cut my arms. I was fed up with this illness and wanted it all to go away but I have to accept that it's here now, maybe forever which sounds quite scary.

This is how it works…

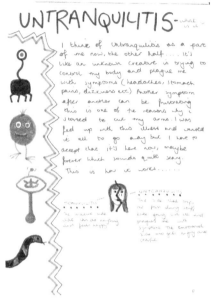

Figure 22

Tranquilitis
The mature side that
can do anything and
feels happy

Untranquilitis
The side that stops me from doing
stuff like going out etc and plagues
me with symptoms. The emotional
side who gets angry and tearful

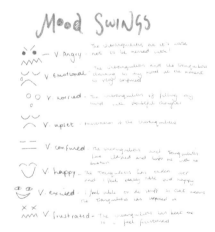

Figure 23

Mood Swings
V. *Angry – the untranquilitis at it's worse – not to be messed with*
V. *emotional – the untranquilitis and the tranquilitis clashing so my mood at the moment is very confused.*
V. *worried – the untranquilitis is filling my mind with doubtful thoughts*
V. *upset – frustration of the tranquilitis*
V. *confused – the untranquilitis and tranquilitis have clashed and leaves me with no emotion*
V. *happy – The Tranquilitis has taken over and I feel really able and happy*
V. *excited – I feel able to do stuff so that means the Tranquilitis has stepped in.*
V. *frustrated – the Untranquilitis has beat me so I feel frustrated*

UNTRANQUILITIS – what is it?

Untranquilitis is a perfect name for this (illness or condition) because

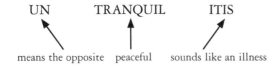

UN   TRANQUIL   ITIS

means the opposite   peaceful   sounds like an illness

Basically the word means an unpeaceful illness, it is not nice to have.

Also each letter stands for a symptom:

U – unable to watch films or TV for
a long period of time
N – no concentration
T – tired all the time
R – really bad headaches
A – abnormal pain
N – unable to make decisions
Q –
U – unable to make decisions
T – interest loss
L –
I – interaction difficulties
T –
I – intelligent with school subjects
but not with life situations
S – switching off.

This is updated from the last time:
When I say updated I mean this is
most of the symptoms I have at the

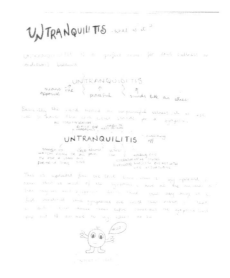

Figure 24

199

moment NOT that they are new symptoms. I don't think that they change it is just sometimes some symptoms are worse than others or that I didn't even notice them before. Sometimes the symptoms just pop out of nowhere to say hello! ha ha

Untranquilitis

Since I've had UNTRANQUILITIS I've been on an emotional roller-coaster. Some days I will feel happy that I have gone to school, I have seen my friends and that I have gone out somewhere but on other days I can feel upset and down mainly because I have done the opposite and I feel sad because I felt I couldn't do it and that I've let UNTRANQUILITIS beat me. And if I can't do it for a couple of days I can reduce to tears, that's why I did the front cover different colours, because each colour represents an emotion.

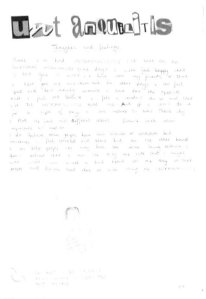

Figure 25

I do believe other people have this illness or condition but sometimes I feel isolated and alone but on the other hand I can help people who may have the same thing because I don't believe that I am the only one with this. I might even write a book about it one day so that people will discover that there is such a thing as UNTRANQUILITIS.

A crying figure with signs
'Do not disturb'
GO AWAY
DO NOT HIDE YOURSELF AWAY.
SPEAK OUT,
YOU ARE NOT ALONE

After this Cathy went through a period when she seemed lower in mood and had been cutting herself. She then spontaneously brought me another book. It was the companion book, 'Tranquilitis'.

Tranquilitis

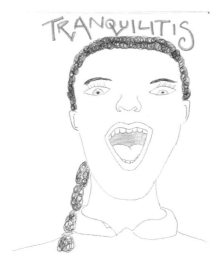

Figure 26

INTRODUCTION

You may think this folder is just like the first one but it's not. In fact it's very different: this explains how good I am on good days and how quickly it can reverse. It also explains about the different switches and how frustrating it can get.

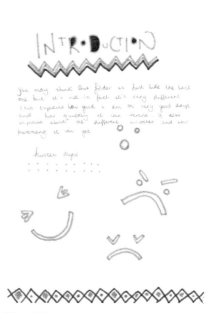

Figure 27

This folder contains:

- DIARY ACCOUNT – Three golden days
- SWITCHING – Different switches
- TRANQUILITIS – What is it?
- + more

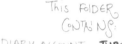

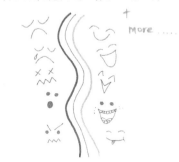

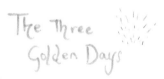

Figure 28

The Three Golden Days
I am going to start a diary from now on, I am going to write down almost everything I do, any symptoms I have and my emotion and mood. It's only a short diary, a three day trial. You will hopefully see the change from untranquilitis – the doubtful, emotional energy one to the nice, kind side of the illness, tranquilitis.

Day 1.
How I feel:

8.10am: I've just woke up in a bad mood for no reason at all I just feel really snappy and don't want anybody nagging me today.

9.05am: should I go to school today? No….. just feel really fed up and frustrated untranquilitis is already stepping in.

Figure 29

9.25am: I'm gonna walk out! I'm going to school I'm gonna walk… erm actually I'm gonna get the bus.

12.30pm: I kept my word, i went to school and yes I catched the bus. Oh… yeah did I mention I walked out of school at 11.30. Oh…no…I didn't but I did get some Science coursework done.

13.45pm: I've done two pieces of Science work and mums still not happy.

15.30pm: My brother has just come home, raced upstairs and went on the playstation 2, hello to you Bruv!

18.30pm: I'm going to watch Halloween H20, I've just had to have our tea round the table I hate it! Don't we get to vote?

22.00pm: I'm going to bed now.

Day 2
How I feel:

8.10am: It's Day 2 and I've just woke up my emotions are balanced for now. I'm going to see Dr Sutton today, I think to suggest going to the learning centre.

9.40: I didn't go to school today but I might go tomorrow. I have got a headache but I think it's because I had a good sleep – I took the Nytol.

12.05pm: My mum is so not fair! She said I'm not allowed to read the newspaper and she keeps taking stuff off me I just wish she'd leave my stuff alone!

2.15pm: I've arrived at home. I've accepted going to the centre instead of the other high school at least everyone will be happier. Aww I still have the headache!

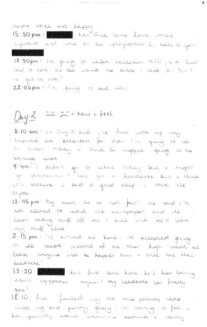

Figure 30

15.30: Bruv has just come home, he's been learning about Egyptians… again! My headache has finally gone!

18.10: Just finished my tea roast potatoes, lamb chops, veg and yummy gravy! I'm starting to feel a bit panicky about tomorrow because I really want to go in tomorrow, but I guess I'll have to see how I feel. I can't predict if untranquilitis or tranquilitis will step in tomorrow but I definitely know which one I'd choose!

9.50pm: I'm going to bed in a minute, I'm a bit anxious about tomorrow but I have to calm down or I won't be able to get to sleep and won't have enough energy for tomorrow anyway!

Day 3
How I feel:

8.15am: A bit happy and a bit sad that I didn't go in <u>AGAIN.</u> When am I just going to be able to go in without doubting? I have a bit of a stomach ache and dizziness.

9.40am: I wanted to go to school today but I have home tuition today anyway.

13.45pm: Mum has took the Sims off me again because I had half an hour of TV. She is not fair!

15.00pm: Just finished my lesson with the teacher, home tuition we did about the RSPCA. Bruv will be home soon the teacher said I seemed happier today.

16.45pm: Mum has finally allowed me on the Sims YESSSS!!!

17.30pm: Just having my tea we are having spaghetti it's gluten and egg free!

19.50pm: I bit calmer today maybe it's because it's no school on Saturday and then it's the holiday.

22.00pm: Going to bed now.

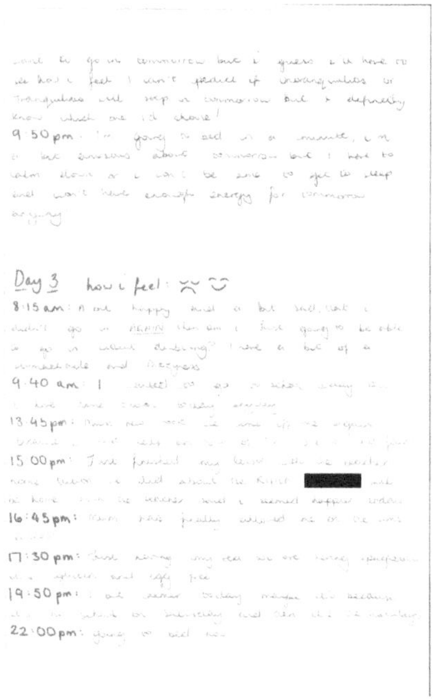

The three golden days
I monitored my emotion, symptoms and how I felt on that day, what I did and what I wanted to do.

Figure 31

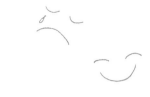

Figure 32

Different Switches

Everything switches around with untranquilitis, the symptoms switch around all the time which is very frustrating, if I decide to go out and then I start to get some symptoms, my emotions switch round too alot so does my mood but that might be because I'm a teenager with lots of hormones! Sometimes I completely switch off and I don't remember things. So if it was something really important to remember the outcome could be dangerous. When I switch off it's like going into a daydream but actually being there in a dream-world. Which means my mind completely forgets everything and anything that I'm doing which is also very dangerous and that I'm not aware of anything.

OFF

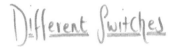

Figure 33

TRANQUILITIS – what is it?

Tranquilitis – what is it?

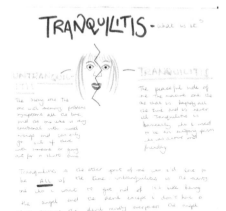

Figure 34

UNTRANQUILITIS
The scary one. The one with memory problems symptoms all the time, and the one who is very emotional with mood swings and can only go out if there with someone or going out for a short time.

TRANQUILITIS
The peaceful side of me. The mature one. The one that is happy all the time and is never ill. Tranquilitis is basically who I used to be, an outgoing person who was active and friendly.

Tranquilitis is the other part of me who I'd love to be <u>ALL</u> of the time. Untranquilitis is the nasty one who I want to get rid of. It's like having the angel and the devil except I don't have a choice because the devil mostly overpowers the angel most of the time.

TRANQUILITIS – what is it?

<u>TRANQUIL</u> <u>ITIS</u>

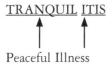

Peaceful Illness

Basically Tranquilitis is the peaceful side of the illness. You can recognise if Tranquilitis or Untranquilitis has decided to step in. It's like having a devil and an angel except I don't have a choice I have to get stick with one or the other.

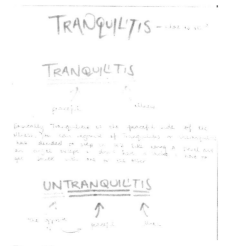

Figure 35

<u>UN</u> <u>TRANQUIL</u> <u>ITIS</u>

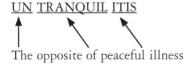

The opposite of peaceful illness

When I go to school I …..
When I go to school I am quite alright I like everything to be in order if anything different happens I get panicky and when I get panicky I think something bad is going to happen so I like to keep my bag and coat close to me, that has my phone, paracetamol and all my other belongings in them so I feel I need to keep my things with me in case my symptoms start and I suddenly have to make an emergency exit. Some days I am okay at school especially with my friends around me I guess because they take my mind off my symptoms and my worries. I do talk

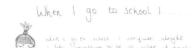

Figure 36

to people at school and have a certain group I hang around with sometimes I wish I could just wave a magic wand and wish my worries and symptoms all away.

Untranquilitis is the doubtful part of me that makes me think I can't achieve goals and do other normal stuff like going out and actually just being able to feel well for once. Tranquilitis is the person who is outgoing the person who I switch too after a few good days and when I'm like this I feel on top of the world! On the other hand, Untranquilitis creeps back in and then I can feel the lowest of low, cutting my arms being frustrated with people and thinking about suicide but I never do because Tranquilitis is still there.

On a good day I …..(Tranquilitis)
On a good day I can go to school as normal, last the whole day, come home smiling. Act mature if I get any symptoms at all. Chill out, go on the Sims, share with Bruv, do homework with Bruv, do chores, go out basically what I used to be able to do.

On a bad day I….. (Untranquilitis)
On a bad day I won't go to school. Answer back to anybody and won't do hardly any work, complain about my symptoms, I'll have really bad symptoms. I won't speak to hardly anyone and I won't go out and get to sleep early enough. I'll also be very emotional and angry with everyone.

When I get frustrated I….
When I get frustrated I get angry with other people easily and I tend to start arguments for no reason. When I get really frustrated about not going to school, not going out somewhere or something else I

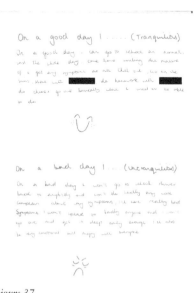

Figure 37

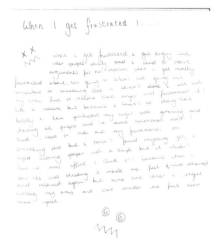

Figure 38

207

haven't done I will cut my arms just to release that anger and frustration it's like a relieve but because I haven't been doing that lately I have projected my anger into groaning and shouting at people and I'm more emotional now. I think I need to take out my frustration on something else but I haven't found anything yet, I tried cutting paper with a knife but it didn't have the same effect. I think it's because when I saw the cuts bleeding it made me feel quite relieved and relaxed again but some time later I regret cutting my arms and that makes me feel even more upset.

Tranquilitis

Thoughts and feelings
I wish that I could be like Tranquilitis all of the time that way I could be a mature person of how I used to be but I can't because sometimes I slip into Untranquilitis and this means trouble! It means mood swings, over-the-top emotions, frustration and anger. So BEWARE.

UNTRANQUILITIS IS HARD TO DEAL WITH BUT AT LEAST I HAVE THE TRANQUILITIS SIDE.

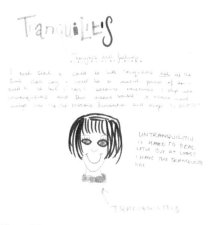

Figure 39

Cathy's description of 'Tranquilitis' and our subsequent discussions continue to have a powerful impact on me.

Tranquilitis is a 'peaceful *illness*'. It is neither a state of *health* nor of simple *peacefulness*. It is not even a state of *peace between the storms*. It is something which gives an *illusion* of peace – another 'trick' is being played. *Tranquilitis* requires vigilance rather than a state of non-pathological, non-complacent surveillance: it still interferes with simple pleasures and 'getting on with life'. It seemed analogous to the 'highs' of bipolar disorder. In bipolar disorder states of misery and elation cannot be equated with ordinary sadness and happiness even if they occur in response to external events. Cathy had no secure emotional base in her body, only experiences of refuge from the storm.

Periods of symptoms interspersed with remissions continued but Cathy was able to go out much more. She attended some courses at a college where the environment suited her better than school. As she approached her 18th birthday I had to transfer her to adult services. Cathy was in two minds. In part it seemed that this was a continuing manifestation of her difficulties with any change. I thought I should attend her first appointment with her to ease the state of transition. I thought she was otherwise highly unlikely to attend.

I also thought that it was a way of communicating directly some of the things she had told me.

I did reflect on whether I was possibly 'acting out in the countertransference'. Might I be *enacting* a parental role rather than *containing* it and holding it in mind with Cathy? I decided that even if I was succumbing to some aspect of this, it was the result of a good appraisal of her developmental needs. I discussed this with my colleague in the adults' psychotherapy service. My colleague accepted my reasons for suggesting this approach and we arranged for me to attend part of the first consultation. I thought Cathy needed this concrete demonstration that I had done all that was reasonable in my role within the mental health services. Cathy agreed to attend on this basis.

Prior to that appointment, Cathy telephoned and asked for an additional appointment with me.

When Cathy came to the consulting room she was silent and remained so for some time. We sat in silence and I observed her. She was now a very tall, slim, striking young woman. As she sat opposite me she stared intently at her finger tips.

Her fingers were long and elegant and she moved them, just touching the tips together. I reflected to myself on how writing and drawing had always been things that Cathy could use to express herself to herself. When she was with people but not actively involved in conversation, she could look like she was somewhere else, on another planet.

I decided to tell Cathy about my observations and reflections. I ended this by saying 'It seems to me that sometimes you live in your fingertips.'

Cathy immediately started talking. She commented on a period of time when she had been much more active, tidying up at home and doing all her own food preparation. She said 'You remember how pleased my parents were? What they didn't realise was that I was only doing my own cooking because I believed it was the only way to make sure I wasn't poisoned.'

I was relieved that Cathy had agreed to attend the department for adults and even more so when she did attend...

10

PARENTS IN PERIL

Is it a parent's rightful place to be in the wrong?

In our work with children and their parents we are present at, and witness to, the origins of later transference phenomena. To be with the baby who is inconsolably crying, to feel his impact and to feel useless and helpless with him and perhaps *for* him can be devastating. So, how much more intense if you are that baby's parents? In the ordinary range of human experiences can anyone make a person feel more intensely than her or his own baby? Can there be any worse experience than seeing your child suffering and be unable to do anything for him?

Winnicott (1956a) described the state of the ordinary devoted mother prenatally and post-natally as *primary maternal preoccupation*. It is a state of particular sensitivity, which builds upon her foundations of personality, to provide the structures which will enable her to attune and adapt to her baby. Holding her baby in mind and body is the first component of the facilitating environment. Kleinian theory conceptualises this as a stage of projective and identificatory processes in the baby emphasising the concreteness with which these may be experienced by the mother in her caring for her child. Other people around the baby are not immune to such processes, particularly when they are in close caring relationships with the baby. The ordinarily devoted father, the involved extended family member and other figures of attachment will all become a particular focus for the child and form bonds through these everyday, highly intense routes of relating.

The processes of parenting produce inevitable challenges for parents. Overall these are likely to build upon their development to date. Parents can find the necessary resources within themselves and may find additional abilities arising in their need to remain functioning for their child. However, at times parents may feel they are being tested beyond endurance. Even with an 'ordinarily demanding and developing baby' their ability to contend with what is evoked may be challenged. Resonances with areas of vulnerability from their own earliest experiences may occur. In conjunction with other challenges, for example complex experiences in labour, illness, sleepless nights, financial worries, stressful relationships or constitutional vulnerabilities, ego-functioning can be adversely affected. Examples occur throughout the book. For example, Mrs T (*Clinical example 1.2*) started with her daughter but 'found' the Devil: when she recovered from her psychosis she was able to start again and determinedly sought to be the mother her daughter needed.

Preconceptions and conceptions

The information to be gained by obtaining mothers' previous obstetric experiences and including a detailed exploration of pregnancy, labour and their start with their baby cannot be underestimated. The mothers whose children presented in 'problems with poo' exemplified this. Operating at a level of secondary, tertiary and quaternary referral I found, almost invariably, complex obstetric histories, for example *Clinical example 6.5* where the pregnancy became a cancer. In other cases obstetric complications such as haemorrhage caused disruption and the potential for death. The process through which the details come to light can be equally informative.

Clinical example 10.1

Jackie was eight years old when referred because of medically unexplained faecal incontinence. She came with both parents and her brother who was four years older. Having gathered various parts of the background history I drew up the family tree using a whiteboard so that we could all see it clearly. During this process Jackie's mother sat still and was fairly quiet, participating less than other family members. When this process appeared to have reached a natural conclusion from the family members' point of view I asked if there was anyone missing.

Children and mother said 'No' but father said 'What about Edie?'

Mr L told me that Edie had been their first child and that she had died of a heart condition at two days old.

When I asked Mrs L about Edie, she came to life. She described how Edie's problems had not been diagnosed immediately. Edie had appeared to be healthy, but then her mother had drawn the nurses' attention to her feeling that something was wrong in her breathing and that she did not seem very warm. The heating in the nursery was turned up. Soon after, Mr L was told that there was a heart problem. Edie was referred straightaway to a specialist hospital but Mrs L was not able to accompany her. Edie died. The funeral directors discussed the possibilities for burial with Mr L who took full responsibility for arrangements. He wanted to spare his wife further upset. They suggested burying her in a coffin with an adult corpse rather than burying her on her own. Mr L agreed.

The whole family became involved in the discussion, parents recounting and the children hearing about this essential part of their life for the first time.

Gathering the raw data of a family tree in terms of constituent members and relevant biomedical data is one outcome of obtaining a family tree. The *procedure* could be completed as a routine factual exercise or via a question-naire, but this could miss the opportunity to capitalise on the clinical value of the *process* through which the information was communicated.

For many parents it may be possible for them to learn to live with the sadness of loss. It can only ever be a gap in their lives. But it does not have to be one which produces a fundamental fault line in family life and cause rever-berations through the subsequent generation. However, if obtaining a family history is restricted to a procedure of gathering only raw data about the 'index' child, it misses other information including obstetric details such as long time-gaps between children, perhaps indicating the absence of longed-for children who were not conceived, not carried through to delivery or who died or were otherwise lost to the parents. Its proper place as part of the clinical process has been missed if it becomes a mere procedure of obtaining data.

Defence or attack: porcupines and parents

Paediatricians may ask for psychiatric involvement where there are manifest physical signs but the response to treatment is not as great as expected. These represent a particular form of 'medically unexplained symptoms and signs'. This may occur with or without other specific concerns about the child. The following case illustrates further the importance of appreciating family context and history and the conscious and unconscious processes of parents in their care-giving.

Clinical example 10.2(a)

Mary was referred when she was two years old. She was well known to the paediatric team because she had had seven admissions since she was three months old: admissions varied in length from 3- 17 days. Each admission had been for treatment of eczema, but 'family problems' had been noted each time. Her speech development was noted as being slightly slow.

Mary lived with her sister (5 years) half-brother (16 years) and her parents Mr and Mrs W: her 18-year-old half-sister lived away from the family. Social Services had previously been involved because of violence from Mrs W to her step-son. There had not been any further violence, but their relationship continued to be very difficult. The background information available from previous child psychiatry involvement also noted that during her pregnancy with Mary, Mrs W had considered a termination of pregnancy: she had also had two ante-partum haemorrhages.

> I met Mr and Mrs W and Mary on the ward prior to discharge to
> arrange to meet the whole family for an outpatient consultation. I was
> struck by how red and raw Mary's skin was, how miserable she looked
> and how agitated her parents appeared.

I used a Milan Family Systems[1] approach, modified because its rigorous
application involves a number of therapists and particular facilities. There
is a particular emphasis on the use of *positive connotation*. This is a clear
statement to each family member highlighting positive aspects of their
involvement in family life. These aspects are less likely to have featured
explicitly or dominantly in contrast to difficulties and conflicts. The positive
connotation is a statement of the perceived intention behind actions, even if
the actions themselves did not have a good outcome. It can initially appear
to be tantamount to a denial of behaviour which can appear, for example,
selfish or authoritarian. However, it can be a powerful acknowledgement of
a component of wishing to do the right thing. From a psychoanalytic point
of view, it serves to capture ambivalence and internal conflict by naming
a beneficial component, even an altruistic wish, however misguided the
manifest behaviour is, or however much ego-centric, destructive or aggressive
feelings may be operating. It captures the possibility of 'Yes and...' rather
than 'Yes but...'. It treats behaviour and behavioural patterns as symptoms
produced by defence mechanisms brought into action by signal anxiety as
a result of unconscious processes (see Chapter 1). It accepts conscious and
unconscious contributions which influence people's abilities to try and do the
right thing.

Clinical example 10.2(b)

I saw the family with a social work colleague. At the start of the consultation, Mary's misery and her parents' agitation were again evident. Her
cry was persistent and whining. Her parents did not respond to her
warmly or handle her gently. They were sharp and unpleasant in their
exchanges with each other seeming to have arrived with an agenda of
blaming rather than addressing problems. Mary's elder sister, Sally, was
friendly to the point of over-familiarity. The children were left to their
own devices except for sharp comments to put them in check when
their behaviour became more raucous. Mary's brother John was absent.

The 'prickliness' between the parents and towards Mary over-rode
my initial attempts to engage them and I found it an extremely difficult
consultation to manage. After about 45 minutes John arrived. He had
been given incorrect directions but he had persisted and eventually

found us. His arrival increased the prickliness. At this point I felt all but overwhelmed by the chaos and antipathy. I felt useless and it took a conscious effort to remind myself that I had training that was specifically to manage such situations. This effort of will did help me 'find myself', to rise to the challenge, rather than to act out the countertransference created in being with this complex family.

What became very apparent was how little time they all spent together as a family. Mother worked long hours, feeling desperate that she must hold her own in what she experienced as a demanding job. Father worked as a clerk, a job he felt was below his potential. He attended evening classes in order to gain qualifications to progress into a professional career. He was very closely involved in the care of the two girls, taking them to school or nursery each morning and spending time attending to them in the evenings, as did their half-brother. John was at college working towards exams and hoping eventually to go to university.

The first interview was spent gathering details of these day-to-day activities. The parents complained of the children being demanding and that this led to further arguments between the parents. The hostility between the parents would readily re-surface and there was mention of the violence there had been by mother to step-son. Mary eventually settled to the extent of becoming simply withdrawn.

The most important shared characteristic of their families of origin was the placing of a high value on determination, which sometimes spilled over into obstinacy. This was one of the complaints both parents made about the children, seeing them often as obstinate and disobedient. Conflicts occurred between Mr X and John; the latter would push this to a certain point but then climb down and obey Mr X. Neither of the two younger children slept well and this would result in disturbed evenings and nights for the parents.

Both parents had come to this country ten years earlier as a result of racial problems in their countries of birth, where they were part of an ethnic minority group which had become the focus of racial and political harassment. Mrs X was the eldest of seven children. She had two children from her arranged first marriage. This marriage, to a man much older than herself, was intolerable for her and she left him, which was unheard of in her culture, taking the children with her. Mr X was younger than his wife. He was the third youngest of thirteen children and the last of the family to leave home, having looked after his elderly widowed mother until his marriage. Marrying a divorced woman was unusual in their culture and there had been family opposition to it.

After a planned break for discussion with my colleague, I returned to find Mary screaming and stripped down to her underwear. Her mother was spreading eczema cream all over her. She had seemed relatively content before, but mother informed us that she had become terribly upset because of her skin itching.

The feedback to the family emphasised just how determined they had needed to be just to get to the meeting, emphasising this for John, and how difficult this immediate meeting had been for all of them. Addressing mother and father we commented on the long hours they worked and studied to provide the best possible home for the family. The children were praised for having learnt the lesson the parents had learnt in their families of origin, i.e. the way to be liked was to be determined or even obstinate. Mary was identified as expressing the way things get under everybody's skin. The children's demanding-ness was seen as stemming from worry about their arguing and being concerned for them, but we accepted that they did not realise that this stopped the parents getting together more. The final remarks were on how hard each of them was working to try and make the family succeed and stay together.

I was taken by surprise how the approach to feedback galvanised all the family members. I had been clear with them that I needed to be able to present my thoughts back to them for their consideration but that their responses would need to await subsequent meetings and would not be discussed immediately. They all listened to what I said, giving it their absolute attention. Mr and Mrs W and John nodded in agreement as I addressed each of them personally.

There were three further family consultations over the next few months, but then they did not attend and did not respond to correspondence. Although the ending was unsatisfactory, there were marked changes. Mary's skin improved dramatically and only minimal amounts of steroid cream were being used. In suffering less from her eczema, there was a primary gain which was added to by the avoidance of adverse secondary effects from having to use topical steroids. She had no further admissions to hospital in the subsequent two years. In addition her speech improved to be within an ordinary range and she was lively and playful. Her parents had also achieved a better balance in their lives and were in less conflict with each other.

Observing and interacting with Mr and Mrs W was a very complicated, difficult, even irritating experience. They were 'prickly'. However, when *I* was able to take a different perspective and manage my countertransference better, *they* behaved differently. The approach placed great emphasis on my need to understand better the factors which were contributing to a situation which was intolerable for all the family members. In conjunction with this it demands appreciation and acceptance without necessarily intellectual understanding that the situation has arisen *despite* the best intentions of the parties involved. Bad situations can arise even in the absence of ill will.

Although the Milan Model is formulated as a treatment derived from systems theory, it can also be understood as a distillate of psychoanalytic ideas, structured in a way which can be applied to the complexity of consulting to whole families. Its structure enabled me to manage my countertransference better, particularly in response to my experience of the family atmosphere as 'prickly'.

My associations to 'pricliness' led me to the image of a porcupine. To come into contact with a porcupine's quills can be extremely painful. At times and in certain societies there has been a belief that porcupines use their quills aggressively, even being able to launch them. However, their quills are their only defence apart from fleeing a situation. In fact, if a threatening figure remains, the threatened porcupine may run backwards, perhaps embedding some quills in the feared figure, leaving it better able to make its escape going forward. The secret of getting to know a porcupine safely is to keep sufficient distance and behave in a way that challenges the porcupine's belief in you as a threat.

Trying … but could do better?

I thought Mr and Mrs W were people who were on the verge of being overwhelmed by the demands of both the internal and the external world. Over and above this, they had moved to a point in their own ego-functioning at which more immature defence mechanisms would 'take charge'. But even these were beginning to fail: they were experiencing 'raw anxiety'. I became able to appreciate that my experience of being with them, which had at times felt overtly hostile, was in fact being with people who were utterly desperate, down to their last-ditch defences (see Chapter 5). This was the 'dynamics of desperation', not entrenched investment in aggression or sadism.[2]

For Mary and her family, other professionals had tried to help before and further difficulties meant that others had to try subsequently. In line with my experience, many found them 'very trying' in the sense of 'straining patience or endurance', 'annoying', 'vexatious'. As a family they *were* trying, trying extremely hard to make a bad situation better. This dynamic operates in many situations, including those where care and/or protection are of such concern that child protection procedures need to be enacted. *Understanding* does not mean that judgements about what is 'good-enough' care are ignored. Children need to be safe and parents are done a disservice if 'not-good-enough' is tacitly colluded with by professionals to avoid challenging them (Sutton 2008 and 2011). Maintaining a *clinical* stance means being prepared to judge if parents are *unable* to provide 'good-enough' care, distinguishing this from a *moral* stance about parents which is the realm of the law not of medicine.

The clinician, the parents and their child's illness

The professional role with parents can be summarised as: (a) assisting parents in the care of their child in order that there can be reasonable expectations of the child (given his emotional state and developmental stage) and of the parents; (b) providing something for the child that the parents cannot (Sutton and Hughes 2005).

Parents bring their own experiences into the paediatric setting which means that transferences arise from them and need to be managed. This can be a very complex area but the key issue in managing it is to remember that the parent is not the patient: we collaborate with parents as adults who have the right to our opinions about the welfare of their children. But those opinions may need to be couched in particular ways to manage unconscious as well as conscious processes.

Parental anxiety: some attributions and misattributions

The opportunities for understanding and misunderstanding conscious motivation and intention in parents' behaviour are innumerable. Changing OUR understanding can be the first step towards parents and children being able to overcome problems which arise in association with physical health concerns. The preceding case describes how I came to understand more about conflict and desperation. Some other common themes will now be explored.

The 'over-anxious parent'

What does it mean when a clinician thinks about or refers to a parent as 'over-anxious'? I think it means that the parent continues to be anxious despite the practitioner thinking she can cease to be so and has given reasons for this that he thinks should be sufficient. The clinician will have *assured* the parent that everything is fine but is more likely to use the word 'reassured' to describe what he did .

But if parents still do not have confidence in their child's safety or health, they cannot be *re*-assured – they have never been *assured*. The clinician has merely confirmed his own confidence and re-emphasised that he does not understand why the parent feels like she does. Achieving progress requires a truly empathic response which acknowledges a parent's state of mind and that the clinician still does not understand it. This may be achieved implicitly through further explanations but can be enhanced by a simple statement of not understanding the parent's continuing anxiety.

Clinical example 10.3

Baby Jason had symptoms and signs which required investigation via cardiac catheterisation. The cardiologist explained the procedure carefully. Jason's mother appeared to understand what was involved and gave her consent.

After the cardiologist left, the mother burst into tears.

The nurse who had attended with the cardiologist refrained from simple reassurance. She asked what was wrong as she had appeared confident about what was going to happen before.

Jason's mother replied that she knew he needed the procedure but 'I don't understand why he has to be castrated.'

The nurse was then able to provide explanation, assurance and reassurance.

In MUS, it can be particularly important to extend the historical enquiry into family members' wider experience of medical care. Asking if there have been previous events which left mistrust of health professionals can bring forward stories of 'near misses' or actual catastrophes. These may have been recent but can have been in the distant past. Listening without being defensive of medical colleagues or making judgements about whether the concerns appear justified demonstrates an approach which seeks to be well-informed rather than partisan. The process separates past and present and can be a vehicle to provide appropriate assurances and facilitate current care.

Beyond anxiety

When progress is not possible, then the possibility of parental mental health problems has to be considered. Problems may range through anxiety states, depression and obsessional disorders to the unusual possibility of delusional beliefs and psychosis.

Preoccupation with the bodily health of a child allied with persistently and insistently seeking medical opinions and procedures is seen in the rare condition 'Factitious Illness' (Lazenbatt and Taylor 2011). It is a form of child abuse in which false symptoms are described and physical signs may be induced. The presentation is not driven by anxiety but by an investment in the relationships and processes involved in child health and illness care. There is a perverse investment in the child's body, and the relationships which can be formed around it are a source of gratification.

Clinicians themselves become unwitting victims through the parent's actions duping them into dangerous unnecessary procedures which may put the child at further risk. Even when not life-threatening, it can be severely damaging for children's mental health to be presented as ill without feeling or being ill. This may even be compounded by a child being made into a hapless 'accomplice', presenting non-existent symptoms or other information. The origins of the parent's psychopathology may be in childhood trauma but the outcome is the establishment of mental processes such as *identification with the aggressor* (Freud A. 1936).

Clinical example 10.4

Rory was four years old. He had haemophilia which had become very difficult to manage. He had been admitted repeatedly but his haemoglobin remained at levels requiring further intervention. There was clear evidence of blood loss but not of the site of this.

His nurses and doctors were concerned for his parents, who appeared attentive and devoted carers. As part of support for them, child mental health involvement was arranged. The child psychiatrist then arranged psychiatric assessment of the parents.

Meanwhile, concerns began to be raised that the parents may be causing bleeding from skin sites and that this accounted for non-healing and blood loss. The suggestion led to differences of opinion among staff – some not believing it possible, others even outraged by the suggestion.

Psychiatric assessment revealed the father's own history which included severe childhood abuse. His relational patterns and antisocial development led to a diagnosis of a psychopathic disorder. Some staff reacted to the use of this term as unfair and wrong.

Child protection procedures ensued during which his parents admitted to causing bleeding.

The responses engendered in staff who 'felt for' the father in his predicament can be understood as partly countertransference. Learning of his childhood mistreatment and neglect amplified this further. But it can be seen that the child's safety relied on this countertransference being understood for what it was. It was essential that the clinical opinion was not confused with a moral judgement. Ultimately, it is also essential to appreciate that we do not serve parents well if we unwittingly compound or collude with their failing care and protection of their children (Sutton 2011).

Metaphor and responding to anxiety

The place of metaphor in everyday life and its value in thinking about MUS developmentally and clinically were described in Chapter 8. Its use in working with parents in MUS has a two-fold application. It can throw light not only on the child's struggle but on that of the parents.

Two common metaphors – *Walking a tight rope* and *On a knife edge* were discussed in Chapter 8. They can be valuable images to use with parents as they capture how delicately balanced they fear the situation is, the sense of dread and threat to bodily integrity which is contained in the symptoms *and* aspects of universal experience. Looking for the metaphor that captures enough for particular parents can be a productive clinical process. It demonstrates an authentic desire to capture the quality and intensity of what is happening for them. This can be extended to the creation of a personal analogy or metaphor which becomes a parental equivalent to children giving a name for their illness. This form of exploration also opens the way to learning more from people of the family culture and general cultural issues that may be influential.

Impediment or advocate?

A frequent comment heard about parents is that they do not let their child speak for himself. The obverse also arises – some parents desperately encourage their child to talk but the child does not speak. The importance of holding to basic principles and articulating them assumes even more importance: (a) we are doctors who will listen if children talk to us but children do not have to talk to us; (b) a child talking or not talking is part of our clinical examination, an observation; (c) a parent talking and a child not talking is an observation.

To develop adequate understanding of a child we require details of whether a behaviour pattern is acute or chronic, constant or intermittent, situational or non-situational. The clinical consultation offers the opportunity to ask about the child generally in their lives and to observe them with their parents. As we engage with what presents to us we may find the child does come to say more or does not; with experience we may have learnt responses which are more likely to mean a child can speak to us. It is only by *not* making the aim of the consultation that the child talks to us that we can make a proper assessment.

Integrating all the information from the history and observation requires circumspection. If we ascribe cause or purpose prematurely we can fail to appreciate the variety of possible reasons. For example, saying that a child *wouldn't talk* is only one possibility when the observation was in fact only that he *did not* talk. Even if a child is known to have the power of speech, he may not be able to use it all the time. The fact that a clinician addresses her enquiry to a child but the parent answers is only an observation: there may be a variety of reasons for it happening. It is possible that a parent may have a conscious wish to prevent the child from speaking. However, it could be that parents and child have negotiated this before coming and the child has asked for the parent to do the talking: a parent may have found from experience that the child cannot readily respond to questioning and try to help by initiating the account or response.

From a psychodynamic perspective, there may be pre-conscious or unconscious triggers from the child to which a parent is automatically responding. By 'pre-conscious' I am mean that the issues may have been conscious previously or may be emerging into a form which it may now be possible to experience consciously. The response of the parent may therefore occupy a space which comes under the heading *'it goes without saying'* which includes that it may not even be fully formed into a thought. The response may in one way be 'thoughtless' but, in the idiomatic sense, it is a very 'thoughtful' i.e. a considerate response. In speaking *for* her child a parent may be a true advocate fulfilling a function for which the child does not at that moment have the necessary resources. It is a continuation of the *auxiliary-ego* function that children may require from their parents. What may superficially appear to be an impediment may actually be the route through which his voice is heard.

These general principles are especially important where there is concern about health and safety. In children with MUS it can be a central issue given the complex constellation of alexythymia/aphorylexia described in Chapter 8.

The place of a parent is in the wrong

The ordinary processes of parenting mean that the primary regular recipient of a child's projections and projective identificatory processes will be their parents. A parent's ability to be a container into which unmanageable mental experiences can be projected and held is a primary function. It persists in varying degrees depending on the child's development and life events.

Parenting relies on a particular form of reflective practice. *Clinical example 5.1* exemplified the importance of a parent being able to contend with her child blaming her for everything. Appreciating that the sense of 'wrongness' has to find a place and to be contained and reflected upon emphasises also why clinicians have to occupy positions of negative capability and negative culpability. This can prevent breakdown of communication and promote a sense of common purpose.

Clinical example 10.5

Mrs B attended consultations with her daughter Yasmin (*Clinical example 8.2*). She tolerated Yasmin's vitriolic verbal attacks but was left feeling that whatever she did was wrong. I explained to Yasmin that I thought the key point she was communicating was the sense of 'wrong-ness'. It seemed the only way to do this was by putting mother

---

in the wrong – the place for the wrong was in her. Mrs B could accept this possibility and it enabled her to maintain her tolerant approach. Simultaneously she still had to avoid 'playing into' anything which might compound this dynamic and make it more likely to take on a life of its own.

Yasmin still needed mechanisms to deal with the fact that 'feeling in the wrong' was actually 'being right' and further twists and turns continued. She continued to need to assert herself by being in opposition.

The paradoxical possibilities of identificatory processes

Identifying with another person can be conscious or unconscious. For adolescents, seeking to look like, speak like and act like their peers or people whom they admire is very much part of the ordinary developmental process. For younger children, engaging in activities they have seen one or other parent doing is usual. These things can be expressions of admiration and aspiration while they cope with the changes inevitable in relationships. The little girl who sits down next to her mother who is breastfeeding and feeds her doll is an example of 'being the mother' to cope with the loss of that previous relationship with the mother. Identifying with and playing with being the parent gives a chance to test out through fantasy in readiness for the reality. The gap which is the loss of the prior relationship becomes a space in which future possibilities can be experienced in play.

Undue reliance on projective and identificatory processes can give rise to difficulties when developmental pressures move towards separation and individuation. This comes to the fore in adolescence. It was evident in Yasmin's 'use' of her mother: as with the parent, so with the therapist. And being human, mistakes will be made by good-enough parents and therapists. The experience of adults finding their limits is one of the essential ingredients for adolescents in finding their own. Winnicott (1963a: 258) captured this: 'So in the end we succeed by failing – failing the patient's way ... [the relationship is] turned into a new dependence in which the patient brings the bad external factor into the area of his or her omnipotent control, and the area managed by projection and introjections...'

Identificatory processes may also give parent and child a rendezvous point, a chance to meet again at a point where they had previously lost each other. This was evident for Vanessa (*Clinical example 7.1*) and her mother. An episode after Vanessa injured her ankle and slipped downstairs (*Clinical example 7.1e*) illustrated one aspect of her mother's reliance on identificatory processes for decision-making.

Clinical example 10.6

Vanessa's symptoms repeatedly challenged her mother to cope with her own uncertainties, to try to find it in herself to cope and have confidence in her ability to care for Vanessa. She had always been open in seeking assistance in how to respond to Vanessa's symptoms, and made explicit her anxieties.

Vanessa developed problems with her elbow as a consequence of other injuries. In the next consultation with them together, her mother was confident and had no anxieties about what to do for Vanessa. I commented on this contrast and asked if she knew what made the difference. Mother was able to reply without any hesitation. She felt she knew exactly what to do because she had had this problem herself and knew exactly what it was like.

Vanessa and her mother were able to capitalise on this process. It did not induce difficulties for Vanessa as it met her needs where they needed to be met without provoking any sense of denial of her individuality – something which might have occurred, for example, for Yasmin. They both grew through this experience: no one lost and everyone gained. This is not always the case.

Clinical example 10.7

Mrs G attended the children's department because of her daughter's severe anxiety. She described how she and her husband both had chronic agoraphobia but that becoming parents had enabled them to make progress. During the pregnancy, they had gradually been able to undertake small trips out, initially together, but then when their daughter was born they went out, apparently, independently.

I asked how each parent managed going out without the other. Mrs G said 'We had the pram to hang on to ... it was a "white-knuckle" ride!'

In this case, both parents' functioning was temporarily enhanced by their new life-stage of parenthood. However, their daughter became an attachment figure for them in their journeys. Despite their best efforts, the child's experience was of being the container for parental anxiety and recipient of 'alien' projections. The foundations were laid for her extremely disabling symptoms.

Parents' own sense of well-being and self-esteem can depend on their children thriving or be enhanced by seeing them develop. Managed sensitively, children's illnesses or problems can be a chance for 'one step back, two steps forward': the child's needs work in the service of both child and parent. There may be new developmental possibilities for parents as they find it in themselves to do new things.

Case example 10.8

Mrs C described with some bemusement how she was managing some very difficult situations in a much different way from usual.

Serious allegations had been made against one of her children and the police had been involved. The child had denied the allegations but was being harassed by the accusers. Mrs C described how she had always previously been prepared to use violence in difficult situations, but that she knew she had to avoid doing so in this situation as it would probably make things worse for her child. Her bemusement stemmed from the fact that she experienced this new way of behaving as something she might not have been able to do, nor perhaps wished to do, previously. Through the care of her child, she found a new sense of herself as someone who could control her violent impulses and wishes.

Mrs C's *splitting and projection into the child in the service of parental ego-functioning* (Sutton and Hughes 2005: 178) was 'ego-syntonic' but took her by surprise because it crystallised a new development in her. To paraphrase and adapt Groddeck (1925: 199), 'have a child and you may find in you the mother you need for your child'.

Clinician's identificatory processes

Inevitably clinicians find themselves dealing with situations with which they are familiar from personal experience. Deciding how to use this in the service of patients and parents requires careful reflection. Having been through *similar events* cannot be equated with having had *similar experiences*. Neither do they equate to needing similar solutions. Identifying with parents may give another vantage point from which to orientate ourselves to their problems but it may mask our inability to see their situation properly. Detailed discussion of self-disclosure from personal experience of children, our own or other people's has many facets and lies beyond the scope of this book. However, I will highlight some points.

If we use something from personal experience, we then have to decide if we make this explicit. Classical psychoanalytic technique proscribes self-disclosure and this remains a general guideline for psychoanalytic psychotherapy.[3] Arguments in favour of disclosure often centre on issues of power. Non-disclosure is viewed as unjust when juxtaposed with the expectation that patients strive for full self-disclosure. I think this misunderstands the nature of the service the practitioner can provide for the patient, or in the present context, the parent. If it does occur as an act of subjugation, then the practitioner has failed either through acting out in the countertransference or being a sadistic anti-therapist.

We cannot *not* be influenced by our experiences, but in translating them into clinical practice we need to ensure we triangulate these with other evidence from clinical experience, research, theory and disciplined reflection on incidental observations. If considering explicitly stating that personal experience or practice is the source of a comment or recommendation, the clinician has to think what this might mean to parents generally and to this parent in particular. To say 'I did this' or 'I felt this' is very different from 'I've seen this/come across this being done...' or 'I've seen situations where parents feel like...' in terms of its potential impact upon them.

If a parent disagrees or rejects what is put forward explicitly as self-disclosure she may fear that she is jeopardising the continuing assistance that she needs. If a suggestion is rejected, is it because it does not seem to be a good idea or will the practitioner experience it as an affront or an attack on their competence? It may even *be* an attack regardless of any validity contained in the suggestion. Alternatively, to act on it may contain a sense of humiliation in that the practitioner is not only able to do this work, she is also a super-parent. Self-disclosure may be as much an acting out of the countertransference or of omnipotence as the resistance to doing so. It may also have a seductive quality – making parent and therapist the same rather than acknowledging the different roles they are in. Powerful feelings which arise between clinician and parent may be split off from the immediate relationship, with the danger that they will be enacted towards the child.

My position is that I do not make it explicit if I am using personal experiences of caring for children. Where I have used them I am guided through the cross-referencing and reflection described earlier. I do not want to place a responsibility on a parent to replicate my actions or inactions by asking them to identify with me as if I am an ideal parent.

Summary and conclusions

Our work with parents re-emphasises the importance of knowing our place in the lives of children. The legal framework within which we practise identifies the paramountcy of children's needs. In the overwhelming majority of children's lives the best people to fulfil their needs are their parents. Only if they are unable to should they be denied that responsibility.

Parents cannot fulfil their child's needs in their entirety; recognising and responding to this is part of good-enough parenting. Where concerns arise about health and illness, clinicians are appropriate adjuncts to the care of children. Conscious and unconscious processes and the high stakes involved in supporting development and bodily integrity can present very specific challenges to both parents and professionals. Due respect needs to be accorded to parents' emotional lives and relationships but clinicians can best manage these by remembering that they are only involved with these parents because of the child patient. This recognition will best manage pressures which arise from parental transferences and clinicians' countertransferences to them. It properly respects our place in their lives and may add significantly to theirs. If we help a parent parent, we help a parent.

11

IS GOOD MEDICINE HISTORY?

If history is written by the victors, we need to ensure patients aren't the victims.

The long-established teaching that clinical history is the foundation of good diagnostics has stood the test of time (Hampton et al. 1975); Peterson et al. 1992 and Roshan and Rao 2000). This book is based on fundamental respect for two aspects of this:

a   the *procedure* of 'history taking' as a clinical skill with its areas of primary focus which direct the clinician towards areas of elaboration and additional exploration
b   the *process* through which the clinician seeks to obtain an accurate history.

The former gives specific information about the patient's health and illness symptoms. The latter provides additional observational information indicating specific topics about which the patient can give information easily or less easily. It also provides information to the patient about the clinician. It may suggest interest or disinterest with the patient's own particular concerns: it may increase or decrease his confidence in the doctor's clinical acumen.

A well-conducted process demonstrates the clinician communicating, acknowledging her role in the patient's life and truly respecting the patient. It means finding out about the different words, phrases or nuances of approach which may be needed in particular relationships at different times. The history is not simply 'taken'. It is sought, and in seeking it the patient learns about the doctor. The patient learns whether or not the doctor is truly learning about him. The history becomes something that is shared.

Is there a future in the history?

Communication skills are fundamental in clinical practice. The history directs the doctor in her approach to the physical examination, ensuring sufficient general overview is taken and directing her towards any aspects which require more detailed attention. This, in turn, directs her thinking towards which diagnostic investigations may be needed from laboratory services, imaging etc. The conduct of the clinical process offers a crucial opportunity to the patient to assess his doctor and the structures within which she works.

There are aspects of this which 'hard-nosed' practitioners may refer to as 'soft' but they are the hard currency of this process. A readiness to explain will complement the ability for sensitive enquiry or information-giving in constructing the most reasonable course along which to proceed. Authentic clinical encounters in which patients feel their concerns are accepted and appreciated make it more likely that a dialogue with a sense of common purpose can be constructed.

The alternative to a clinical approach which gives a live demonstration to patients of a willingness to put oneself forward for scrutiny and appraisal is that patients place a simple trust in the organisations and institutions which sanction the clinician in her role. To some extent this is inevitable and probably desirable since the technical judgements being made are highly complex. But taken to extreme it would mean that this trust is indiscriminate. It would require patients to accommodate the institution rather than it being a dynamic process through which individualised care can be provided.

The patient's appraisal of the doctor's trustworthiness may be held in abeyance, particularly in emergency situations. Judgements may require further experience as he comes to realise how his own emotional state or the novelty of the situation coloured the picture he had formed of her. The parents in the Surgical Special Care Baby Unit (Chapter 3) described how they became better able to judge which doctors or nurses were more or less adept at different procedures. It also became apparent that as the babies and their parents became more 'long term' and less acutely needy in terms of technical aspects of medical or nursing skills, the 'fit' between parents and staff members became more important irrespective of any acceptable range of variation in technical aptitude.[1]

In extremes, actions which can feel abrupt or tantamount to bullying may be necessary to protect life, limb or function. How these processes are handled, including acceptance of being called to give an account to the patient, will be decisive in the care that can be provided in the future. Helen (*Clinical example 5.1*) was able to engage with all of us involved in her care not only because of how we acted in preparation for and during procedures, but also because we were able to talk together about it afterwards. The process of reflection with patients, a clinical 'reminiscing 'with them, can allow anger, fear and any associated sense of shame about behaviour to be processed. There is less likelihood of inducing further feelings of vulnerability or humiliation, avoiding the emergence of defensive processes which may undermine the patient's ability to contend with subsequent medical care. A clinician may only have appeared to play, or feel she played, a walk-on part in a clinical drama but become an ever-present participant in the future care of one or many patients. It may also be decisive in reducing adverse effects (e.g. medical negligence claims) consequent upon actual or perceived failures of a technical nature. Those instances where medically unexplained symptoms are associated with previous bad experiences may be reduced or more readily managed.

For psychoanalytic practice, becoming part of the patient's living history and life is the method and medium of assessment and diagnostic formulation. It may also become the route through which the still-present traumatic effects of past experiences can be overcome. Ghosts can be laid to rest, and dragons can be tamed. When this is not possible they may still be better accommodated and their adverse effects cause less disruption to the equilibrium and equanimity of patients and the key people in their lives.[2]

But what is 'good medicine'?

In the UK, the General Medical Council (2006) provides guidance for doctors in the document 'Good Medical Practice' (GMP). In this present context, I want to consider three issues in particular:

- *Make the care of your patient your first concern*
- *Protect and promote the health of patients and the public*
- *Be honest and open and act with integrity*
  – Never abuse your patients' trust in you or the public's trust in the profession.

In giving primacy of place to the patient's welfare, the General Medical Council establishes the centrality of the need for a patient's experience of clinical encounters to be authentic, i.e. necessarily and essentially about *him*. However, a 'clinical encounter' as I have described cannot simply be considered an event; it is a process which may be short-lived or unfold over many years. Judging its 'authenticity' may not rely on satisfaction with all aspects of what happens or with the actual outcome but it does rely on an iterative process which seeks to capitalise on opportunities for building on good experiences and minimising the adverse effects of bad ones.

Clinical example 11.1

Ms J's child had been permanently removed from her care. I had carried out a child psychiatric assessment which contributed to the court proceedings. In conjunction with the social worker's report, my recommendation had significantly contributed to the decision.

I offered to see Ms J to discuss my report after the legal proceedings had been completed in order that she could question me herself rather than only through the cross-questioning by her lawyer. She accepted. When she came, she was interested in and accepting of my assessment and recommendations. There was no sense of animosity or antipathy towards me. But Ms J was furious with the social worker.

I was puzzled by her apparently thoughtful acceptance of me and her vehemence towards the social worker. I had worked very closely with the social worker and Ms J knew this. She also knew I had come to the same conclusions as the social worker. I pointed this out and asked why she had such different views of us.

'You were just doing your job', she said. 'That social worker just had it in for me.'

I had no reason to believe that the social worker had been acting unprofessionally – against the mother rather than for the child. Whatever conscious distinctions Ms J may have offered to account for discriminating between us in this way, I thought there were unconscious mechanisms putting me in the right and the social worker in the wrong. This meant that an integral task of the consultation was to challenge, or at least explore, the basis for what was happening. Both idealisation and denigration are failures of discrimination. If I had explicitly or implicitly confirmed one or the other through word or action, I could have perpetuated or compounded a process which would make Ms J more vulnerable in any future interactions. This was not in an attempt to persuade Ms J to a particular view since she might have construed an attempt to do that as a dismissal of her having a mind of her own – an undermining of her autonomy of thought.

Clinical example 11.2

Mrs Q and Hailey lived alone. They were attending the child psychiatry clinic because of severe difficulties in their relationship. Assessment had led on to treatment consisting of individual psychotherapy for Hailey and concurrent parenthood psychotherapy for Mrs Q.

It became apparent that Mrs Q's ability to care for Hailey was severely impaired to the extent that it constituted emotional abuse which was compounding Hailey's emotional difficulties. The assessing team thought it unlikely that there would be sufficient change in her abilities while they were living together. Child protection procedures led to care proceedings, and the psychiatrist in the team, Dr Y, contributed to these, recommending that Hailey was removed from her mother's care. Mrs Q did not want Hailey removed from her care but did maintain contact with her therapist in the clinic despite this.

A considerable time later, after Mrs Q's contact with the clinic had ended, a mother whose child had been referred for assessment and was due to be seen by Dr Y told the interviewing child mental health practitioner that she was a friend of Mrs Q. This mother knew what had happened but was not concerned about Dr Y's involvement because Mrs Q had told her, 'He can come across as a bit abrupt at times, but he knows his stuff.'

Mrs Q was left with the feeling that there was common purpose in the clinical process with Dr Y. She respected that he had applied himself to her daughter's needs. Differences of opinion had been tolerated without this signifying that opinions were being dismissed: this ability was as important in Dr Y as it was in Mrs Q. They achieved a consensus of what they agreed and disagreed about. This was less likely to undermine future clinical contacts, or at least to minimise any adverse effects. In this particular instance the achievement was as much in the service of the child of Mrs Q's friend as anyone else.

Appreciating that 'consensus' can mean agreement about what is disagreed about (sometimes referred to as *dissensus* [personal communication Fulford K. W. M. 2005]) is an essential element of true respect for patient autonomy and clinical autonomy. Working with children is particularly challenging in this respect since practitioners are always involved with at least one other party in addition to the patient. Since the care of that patient is essentially dependent on that other party, that relationship must be one of necessary and sufficient trust. Managing areas of agreement and disagreement whilst avoiding appearing to be or actually being in alliance with one against the other can be extremely taxing and requires considerable expertise (see *Clinical example 10.2* and *10.4*).

Clinical autonomy revisited

Principled autonomy (Stirrat and Gill 2005) as an ethical framework builds on Gillon's 'four pillars' (Gillon 1985: 60–6). Respect for autonomy as a general principle came into even sharper focus to counter perceived discrepancies of power in clinical interactions. Medical paternalism was seen to have adverse effects, at its extreme building institutions that operate on a denial of individuality and the right to autonomy (Goffman 1961). At the other extreme, patient autonomy could produce a position of apparent absolute right to choose a treatment and an absolute responsibility upon a clinician to provide that treatment if they were capable of delivering it. The clinician's view of whether it is safe or reasonable treatment would be irrelevant. Principled autonomy provides a refinement of the framework to balance competing expectations and demands.

For most people, the clinical care they receive is provided within a framework that places constraints upon what can be done despite the extent of medical knowledge. Insurance companies, charitable organisations and state health services operate within the financial constraints upon them. Treatments which will or will not be available may be explicitly defined or special pleading may be needed in specific instances. If 'clinical autonomy' were only to be defined as the clinician doing what he wants then such constraints could be viewed as an absolute undermining of this principle. However, any clinician operating on such a definition is likely to come into conflict not only with patients, colleagues and health care managers, but also with the law and reality.

To respect a patient's autonomy is to accept fully his right to determine what we as clinicians will or will not proceed with in being involved in his life. That this is not an absolute right is conceptualised in the idea of *mental capacity* (see HMG 2005). There can be states of conditional autonomy (Sutton 1997: 29) in which contingencies apply which mean that the right to self-determination may be affected temporarily or permanently in one or more areas of life. Clinical autonomy can sometimes mean stating emphatically that we cannot be of use even if the patient is urging us to be involved and to do something. The patient's request amounts to her giving consent to have something done, but this may be for reasons which the clinician views as mistaken, ill-informed or in the case of conditions such as dysmorphophobia[3] as 'illness-informed'. We may have to insist that we will not agree to the request if we believe it is harmful or not clinically indicated. Except in extremis, any clinical plan has to consented to by more than one person: a patient or person legally mandated to give assent *and* a clinician.

O'Neill (2002b) crystallises a critical point about rights and responsibilities. Rights can only flow from there being someone with a responsibility to fulfil that right. Responsibility can only be accepted or delegated if the person charged with such responsibility has the resources to act to fulfil it. The corollary is that 'health' cannot be a right because it is beyond anyone's power to ensure it. *Health care* becomes a right when the human, material and structural resources are available. The absence of trained surgeons, medicine, vaccines, bandages etc. direct the argument of responsibility away from the clinical encounter towards resource allocation.

Clinical example 11.3

Patrick had an established psychotic illness. It was agreed by him, his parents, his social workers and the psychiatric team that he was not safe living at home and needed admission to hospital. No hospital bed was available.

Procedures had been agreed in such a situation that adolescents were to be admitted to social services' accommodation until a hospital admission was possible. However, the social work team manager was angry about this and directed her anger towards the psychiatrist. She told him she thought the 'Health Authority' was failing severely in their responsibility.

The psychiatrist said he agreed, pointing out that he was a consultant clinician not the 'Health Authority' and had been pointing out the failure for many years.

So, what is the place of 'patient autonomy' or 'clinical autonomy' in wider institutional processes? Patient and practitioner cannot simply decide on something being a reasonable course of action unless there is this other form of authorisation. In such a situation, it seems to me that the essential element in sustaining authentic clinical encounters is that clinicians must have the authority and autonomy to state the bounds within which they are operating. Patients need to know if they are being seen by a medical student, a junior doctor or a senior doctor. Similarly, they need to know if the doctor's ability to act is constrained not by their own technical capabilities but by the resources made available or actions sanctioned.

In summary, patients need doctors to have *clinical autonomy* to make their assessment of their presentation without unreasonable constraints, to give an account of their understanding of these to their patients, define the facilitating and constraining influences on providing treatment and formulate a plan of action on this basis. Such a position allows doctors to properly define and describe their place and usefulness in patients' lives. It makes it possible for them to be considered trustworthy.

'NICE' or 'NICHE': everything in its place

The illnesses and diseases it is possible to treat have increased exponentially. Advances in medical genetics now make it possible to give extensive accounts of likely future disorder even when no physical symptoms or signs are present. However, even the wealthiest countries cannot make all that is possible available to all who might benefit. In England and Wales, the National Institute of Health and Clinical Excellence has been established to provide guidelines for assessment and care in the National Health Service. The Institute is more commonly referred to as 'NICE' perpetuating its previous title of National Institute for Clinical Excellence. It issues clinical practice guidelines (National Institute for Health & Clinical Excellence 2009b) which are 'systematically developed statements that assist clinicians and patients in making decisions about appropriate treatment for specific conditions' (National Institute for Health & Clinical Excellence 2009a: 10). They are derived from the best available research evidence, using predetermined and systematic methods to identify and evaluate the evidence relating to the specific condition in question. Where evidence is lacking, guidelines incorporate statements and recommendations based upon the consensus statements of a Guideline Development Group but '[They] are not a substitute for professional knowledge and clinical judgement' (National Institute for Health & Clinical Excellence 2009a: 11). This acknowledges the continuing need to allow freedom for individual care to be negotiated between clinicians and patients. However, it is also expected that guidelines nationally will lead to protocols being developed locally (National Institute for Health & Clinical Excellence 2009a: 12). The distinction between *guidelines* and *protocols* is considered below.

The word 'nice', used as an adjective, has 14 different definitions used variously through the years. They range from 'foolish, stupid, senseless' through to 'finely discriminative 'and 'requiring close consideration because not obvious' and 'agreeable, pleasant, satisfactory, delightful, generally commendable'. With such a variety of uses over time it is a word for all seasons ... and perhaps none!

In terms of the distinction between guidelines and protocols, *nice*, in the sense of *finely discriminative*, judgement is required. *Guidelines* describe general principles to help implement and develop practice and policies: a *protocol* is to establish rules to be followed. A crucial distinction in clinical practice is that to step outside a protocol will require a more exceptional defence than being seen to breach a guideline since the permissible scope for interpretation is less. One effect is that a protocol obviates the need for acceptance of the same degree of responsibility on the part of practitioners. In exchange, constraints upon freedom of negotiation with individual patients have to be accepted. It may promote *defensive* as opposed to *defensible practice* (Tan, Sutton and Dornan 2010).

In further exploring the language used, the terminology of *clinical excellence* invites examination, although it deserves a much wider exploration than is possible here. Clinical excellence cannot be other than a 'good thing', a virtuous aspiration. A clinically excellent service would have the highest possible levels of staff, skilled and knowledgeable in the sciences and arts of clinical care; there would be state-of-the-art equipment and the resources and relationships available to meet the needs of all those who may need them. Given that this is not possible for all, what it is reasonable to expect is that we have services that can present themselves authentically, acknowledging their human, technical and financial limitations, i.e. good-enough services which will need planned maintenance, support and development, without losing sight of what would be desirable.

The processes with which organisations such as NICE are concerned are beyond the clinical. They involve issues that demand ethical debate and discourse. The quality of life and the values upon which policies will be formulated and implemented are moral issues. These organisations are involved with decisions about the priority that health and illness care take in the wider social, cultural, political and financial world. NICE is in fact NICHE, a National Institute for Clinical and Health Economics. To describe it as such is not to diminish it but to respect it as an essential component of the overall structure with its own bounds of autonomy, authority and accountability. But to lay claim to a defining role for 'clinical excellence' exceeds these boundaries.

Medicine is too important to be left to doctors

Medical science can describe what can and cannot be done. Medical statistics can provide a framework for quantification which can be structured, analysed and interpreted. Epidemiologists can describe groups and these can inform decisions about populations, but the medical discipline of Public Health cannot tell us about the health and illness needs of individual members of the public. What the possibilities they describe may mean for the *quality* of an individual's life is not the preserve of medical specialisms. These meanings are about other aspects of 'the stuff of life'. Judgements about morality, personal preferences and justice require knowledge from the perspectives of other disciplines and from the public. Doctors may become more knowledgeable in these areas but it is in addition to their specialist medical training and expertise.

Doctors do have an essential contribution to make to this discourse. Some may have particular personal qualities and training: they may have taken the opportunity to learn from their patients if they have been with them through sickness and health, for example doctors who have gained expertise through treating X number of *people* with a disease in contrast to those who have merely seen X *cases* of the disease. This requires opportunities 'to be with' rather than only 'to do to'. These clinicians have accompanied patients in their journey rather than simply coming across them on their journey; they will have additional insights into the quality of these people's lives.

Perverse incentives

GMP includes measures to prevent patients being exploited, for example financially, sexually or for other personal gain. Placing medical care within wide institutional, organisational and political contexts gives rise to other possibilities for exploitation.

As a child psychiatrist working in the National Health Service, hearing someone mention 'breach/breech' was almost always likely to indicate the latter – the obstetric condition of a baby presenting bottom-first rather than head-first in the womb. For most of my career I did not hear it very often. Latterly I have heard it frequently, but with the meaning 'breach' to indicate that a patient has waited longer than a target waiting time, for example four hours in an emergency department or 18 weeks for an outpatient clinic appointment. The percentage of patients achieving this target time was used as a measure of the quality of clinical services.[4] Word of a breach mobilises multiple individuals, clinicians and non-clinicians, in managerial roles. Such has been the importance of targets that ingenious methods, unrelated to the welfare of any patient, were devised to avoid breaches. This process was called *gaming*.[5]

I do not see it as a virtue nor an aspiration to keep patients waiting but unless services could be infinitely and immediately extendable, then this is inevitable unless vast resources are held in reserve when unpredictable peaks of need occur. To hold so much in reserve when there is so much unmet need does not seem financially viable or morally defensible.

The targets set were indiscriminate across different clinical services in the NHS. The particular needs and demands for a service and the resources available to respond were not a factor in establishing the figure. To set throughput of patients as a primary standard for judging clinical care is no more intellectually defensible than criticising producers of a popular chair for not being able to respond quickly when the raw materials are not available. Even if raw materials become available there may be no additional people available and trained to produce the furniture – why not use untrained people and take your chances on the quality? Perhaps produce a different product but issue a report defining this product as the aspirational standard, for example four legs good; two are better.

Achieving a target may mean levelling-down standards in clinical processes. Attention is directed away from the primary task, patient care. Adherence to achieving political and managerial targets and gaming redirect the focus from the patient to the interplay between who will win and who will lose in trying to attain them. It forgets that the biggest losers could be the patients who receive a sub-standard service as much as those who do not receive a service at all. This process is analogous to one of the deviant or distorting developmental processes described earlier in the book. States of mental experience or qualities in relationships can become *cathected*. Rather than being a side-effect to the ego-functioning and development which may give satisfaction or dissatisfaction, advantage or disadvantage, they become ends in themselves. They take on a life of their own, take precedence over healthier functioning and become something to attain: they can become perverse incentives contributing to major failures of care.[6]

Good professional practice requires that doctors resist such processes if they are to remain people in whom vulnerable people can have trust and confidence. To be a knowing, willing participant in such a process should lead a doctor to ask himself if he is in danger of a breach of the GMC's guidance (2006a) to 'Be honest and open and act with integrity … act without delay if you have good reason to believe that you or a colleague may be putting patients at risk… Never abuse your patients' trust in you or the public's trust in the profession.' To be preoccupied with what one is not doing and cannot do may undermine what one can do and engender unrealistic expectations of oneself. It can lead to grave consequences for the health of all parties. Doctors have not been immunised against this.

Pathways, conveyor belts and distribution centres?

Care pathways are algorithms describing anticipated trajectories or ranges of trajectories.[7] Reading about them can become complicated as some are frameworks for population-based service provision while others aspire to be a basis for planning care for an individual. Used properly they can give rise to the question 'What makes this person's needs the same as/different from the anticipated range?' They may make it possible to identify where service changes are needed. They may help professionals orientate differently to the person in front of them as a result of recognising individuality. Used poorly they may be mechanisms which deny variations in the courses of illnesses and the individuality of people. If this results in the formulation of the needs of individuals in terms of services available rather than acknowledging matches and mismatches, they can become a form of 'institutionalisation without walls'.

The ever-increasing cost of medical care does bring even more need for good management systems. The search for these has quite correctly meant finding out what can be learnt from other complex organisations, for example the *Toyota management system*.[8] Supermarket models of sourcing, distributing and retailing have also featured. But their outcome measures are far more readily identified than measures of what constitutes living reasonably through health and illness. Used inappropriately, care pathway models are industrial models applied to non-industrial processes. People are not commodities and unlike patients, cars and carrots tend not to have an experience of their journey.

Harrison (2009) suggests that the adherents of a Biomedical Model have made it far more possible for commodification of health and illness care. Its superficial linearity and reduction of complexity make it attractive as a way of breaking up an overall process into isolated components or procedures for which simpler outcome measures can be described. This serves to limit the likelihood of individual variations in practice, reducing both the need for individuals to accept responsibility and their opportunities to learn from experience.

Menzies Lyth (1960) used psychoanalytic theory to observe, explore and to consult to institutions and organisations. In one of her classical studies she was engaged by a paediatric ward concerned about their failure to retain staff they trained. In this paper she described how interactions resulted in patient care being compartmentalised into procedures. Rather than experiencing continuity of care, patients experienced parts and functions of themselves being attended to. Staff did not experience continuing to care for patients and in consequence were dissatisfied: this discouraged trainees from staying after qualification. She concluded that the structures which emerged to deal with the conscious and unconscious anxieties inherent in the work were counterproductive.

A corollary from the work of Menzies Lyth and subsequent findings from organisational consultancy is that the structures and procedures of institutions need to emerge to equip the staff to perform the primary task of patient care and in continuing to feel able to perform this task. To provide proper care for patients, practitioners need to be treated respectfully in integrating their experiences. This includes taking account of the particular and sometimes peculiar pressures which arise from transference and countertransference phenomena. These phenomena can be the spanners in the works, the grit in even the best-oiled machine and the causes of overheating in the system. This task could be couched as 'looking after them' or in more hard-nosed terms as 'servicing your investment'.

Is good medicine history?

The argument I have been presenting through this book is that there are aspects of good medical care which fundamentally rely on continuity of the experience of being cared for and continuity in providing care. The patient's historical account of their symptoms, contextualised in their life history, is a major signpost to diagnosis. Clinicians respond to this with directed examination and investigation which usually clarifies the possible and probable causes and diagnoses. A patient's experience of this may fundamentally influence the accuracy of the raw data which the doctor can gather. It can affect the extent to which a patient can make good use of what clinicians can provide. Achieving diagnostic clarification and establishing treatment can depend upon knowledge of subtleties and nuances in patients, their carers and their clinical staff. These may be major influences which will only be identifiable through the history patients and doctors develop together.

Good medical practice (General Medical Council 2006b) asks that doctors be aware of patients' future needs and the needs of future patients. This means hearing about the processes of health and illness, seeing their impact on patients and on clinicians through a range of experience of need and absence of need. If not all doctors, then at least a sufficient cohort of doctors, bearing witness to the unfolding of patients' lives, through 'patient-hood' and with awareness of their lives in 'non- patient-hood', will always be needed to provide care and to help in the planning of care and services. They must be supported in assimilating and processing the consequences of their engagement with their patients.

It may be that *good medicine* becomes a version or caricature of the Biomedical Model. This may serve well for financial masters and mistresses preparing the bottom-line or politicians pursuing re-election. Perhaps it will become defined through a superficial lip-service to the tenets of a Biopsychosocial Model whilst the process of care in relationships is depersonalised into procedures in which practitioners are mere mechanisms for protocol-fulfilment. If so, the common humanity which underpins what I consider to be good medical care and which I need as a patient will be lost – good medicine will be history.

NOTES

Chapter 1

1 Mother of Nathan, a 12-year-old patient.
2 Dwayne's treatment is described in Sutton (2001b).
3 Elizabeth's treatment is described in Sutton (1987).

Chapter 2

1 The explanation of the child psychiatrist's role used as an introduction for children by Dr Susanna Isaacs Elmhirst (1921–2010).
2 Also features as *Clinical example 5.3*.
3 Lain-Entralgo P., *El diagnóstico médico* (Barcelona: Salvat, 1982). Cited in Mezzich (2002).
4 *Tentorium*: a membrane separating the areas associated with higher brain functioning from the cerebellum and spinal cord. Hence, 'supratentorial' indicates a view that the problem is with diminished functioning in the mind not the body.
5 A silly or inept person (Shorter Oxford English Dictionary).

Chapter 3

1 Speaker at a workshop discussion during the 10th Ottawa Medical Education Conference 2002.
2 See Chapter 4 for an example of how a 'too-complete' understanding expressed prematurely can be problematic.
3 I am implicitly linking the terminology here to Gillon's descriptions of the types of autonomy as 'autonomy of thought, will and action' in Gillon (1985: chapter 10).
4 Initially at the Royal Free Hospital, London at the request of Dr Dora Black who supervised the programme and subsequently at St Mary's Hospital for Women and Children in Manchester.
5 Freud captured some of the complexities of this from the point of view of psychosexual development in describing the Oedipus complex. Subsequently, psychoanalytic theory has extended this understanding from the classical Oedipal phase (three to five years) to consider its earlier developmental significance. See Laplanche and Pontalis (1988: 282–7).
6 See articles and correspondence in the *British Medical Journal*, January–February 2011 (Fewtrell et al. 2011; Martyn 2011; Renfrew, McGuire and McCormick 2011; Wright 2011; Williams and Prentice 2011).
7 For an analagous discussion of this in relation to doctors' adherence to child protection guidelines see Sutton (2011).
8 There is an extensive literature on using systems theory and psychoanalytic theory in this way. A good starting point is Obholzer and Roberts (1994) and Menzies Lyth (1988).

Chapter 4

1 David Livingstone (1813–73), explorer.
2 For descriptions of these types of conditions see the website of Boston Children's Hospital/Harvard Medical School, http://www.childrenshospital.org/az/Site2187/mainpageS2187P0.html (accessed 26 October 2011).
3 Walsh et al. (1992) remain cited as the reference guidance, e.g. see Johns Hopkins University Dept of Paediatric Urology,http://urology.jhu.edu/pediatric/diseases/DEx2.php (accessed 26 October 2011).
4 *Challenging behaviour*: 'a descriptive concept, […] largely socially constructed, and its meaning is subject to changes in social norms and service delivery patterns over time and across geographical areas. The term itself carries no diagnostic significance, and makes no inferences about the aetiology of the behaviour. It covers a heterogeneous group of behavioural phenomena … Challenging behaviour may be unrelated to psychiatric disorder, but can also be a primary or secondary manifestation of it' (Xeniditis, Russell and Murphy 2001: 109).
5 See 'Skin' in Hinshelwood (1989: 426–30).
6 The theoretical basis of this formulation and a broader explanation will be described in Chapter 6.
7 There are six groups: (1) sex chromosome constellations other than XX or XY; (2) altered hormone production; (3) altered responses of the body to the hormones which bring about sexual differentiation; (4) altered patterns of exposure to hormones during pregnancy; (5) hormonal influences and responsivity in utero leading to abnormalities of the male urogenital tract; (6) children with traumatised genitalia. See Sutton and Whitaker (1998).
8 Surgery took place in various stages. Testes had formed and were located inside the abdomen. There is a significant risk in these situations that cancerous change can occur. The recommendation would have been for their removal even if Lesley had wished for them to be retained. Her penis/clitoris was reduced in size and a vagina was formed. Treatment with feminising hormones also commenced.
9 See Chapter 6 on 'cathexis'.
10 Lest Freud's formulation appears far-fetched consider the following: 'the reality is that when most scientists get up in the morning and stand in the shower and think […] I need to get to work quick because I need to do something, … it's because I just want to sneak a look up mother nature's skirt and see how much stuff I can see, it's just the thrill of discovery'. (Murray 2011).
11 The *manifest content* of a dream refers to the conscious aspects the person has on experiencing and recounting it. However, Freud postulated that there are multiple other components which can be understood through deeper consideration and knowledge of the dreamer's mental life and earlier life experiences. The latter represent the *latent content*. See Freud S. (1927) Dreams. Chapters 5–15.
12 For definitions of sexual and gender identity see Sutton and Whitaker (1998: 156–7).

Chapter 5

1 John Lennon (1940–80).
2 A general point emphasised in my training by Dr Sebastian Kraemer.
3 The dynamic described is at the root of Winnicott's formulation of the 'true self' and the 'false self' which will be referred to in Chapters 7 and 8.
4 Definition of *participative emergence of form*: 'The process by which the various constituents of a complex system contribute to the maintenance or change of that system. The influence of one part of the system may have effects on the whole which appear disproportionate

(greater or lesser) to their actual relative size. The resultant form may or may not be that which was intended' (Tan, Sutton and Dornan 2010).

5 ICD–10 F44.6 Dissociative anaesthesia and sensory loss (World Health Organisation 2007).

6 Anna Freud (1965: 53) suggested that 'a classification of the defence mechanisms according to position in time inevitably partakes of all the doubt and uncertainty which even today attach to chronological pronouncements in analysis. It will probably be best to abandon the attempt so to classify them and, instead, to study in detail the situations which call for the defensive reactions.' However, in a subsequent paper (Freud A. 1970) she did attempt linkage of diagnostic categories and mental mechanisms.

7 See *Psychoanalytic Psychotherapy* (2009) Special Issue: Depressive Disorders in the Life-Cycle: Biology, Environment & Internal World.

8 In using the word 'madness' I accept that I may open myself to criticism that the language we use may distort the proper appreciation and respect for the patient's needs given that it is associated with prejudice. However, it has proven useful so far when properly explained.

9 The ease of making mistakes when moving between individual and population statements is emphasised by Kendall et al.'s paper (2011: 1167) which states '*once a person has self harmed the likelihood that he or she will die by suicide increases 50 to 100 times*' (my emphasis). For this to be correct, it would mean that the act itself would increase the likelihood of committing suicide. This causative or cumulative effect is not indicated by the findings which are cited. If all other things are equal, there is no evidence of more or less likelihood.

Chapter 6

1 Yorkshire Dales saying.

2 I use the word 'divergent' rather than 'deviant' because of its neutrality in moral terms.

3 See Lewin (1992) for an introduction to complexity theory from which this formulation is derived.

4 There are many forms of consultative and supervisory roles. More usually in psychoanalytic circles the term 'consultation' would indicate meeting with staff groups to consider their work from a psychodynamic perspective without having direct clinical contact with patients. My work developed in this way partly driven by resource issues but also through the way in which it was possible to construct a manageable and disciplined role combining different components. It might usefully be called *participative consultation* to acknowledge its difference from other approaches to consultation.

5 See Terry, *Clinical example 1.8*.

6 Transference cure: Symptom improvement which can only be maintained whilst treatment is in progress because the improvement in ego-functioning is dependent on a continuing relationship with the therapist.

7 See Abram (1996) 'Being (continuity of)' and other indexed references.

8 Hirschprung's disease is a dysfunction of the large intestine in which the nerve supply to a section is absent leading to the absence of muscle movement in that section bowel. It is a congenital condition.

9 At that time it was not sufficiently accepted that domestic violence was a child protection issue so no further steps could be taken. See Sutton (2008).

10 A hydatidiform mole is a rare mass or growth that forms inside the uterus at the beginning of a pregnancy (PubMed Health 2010).

11 For ease of exposition throughout the chapter I have used 'sphincter' to denote the aspect of the muscle activity which can come under voluntary control: there is an involuntary component which cannot resist defecation.

Chapter 7

1 The material is included in Sutton (2001a).
2 See Chapter 1 for description of *projection* and *projective identification*.
3 See for example Kraemer (1983).
4 Attributed quotation but perhaps apocryphal.
5 Summarised by Holmes (2011a): 'The majority of children have a favoured "object" to which they turn when stressed or sleepy … [it] is "transitional" in that it bridges the borderland between "me" and "not-me", safely containing children's desires and projections. With its nostalgic maternal resonance, [it] comforts and distracts when the parent is absent, helping the child to forge an independent sense of self… Psychotherapy is "learning to play": re-establishing transitional space in a traumatising and unresponsive world.'
6 See Abram (1996: 311–26).

Chapter 8

1 Susanna Isaacs Elmhirst (1921–2010) made this comment during supervision when I was her trainee, 1982–5.
2 Complexity theory adds weight to Groddeck's exposition of underlying processes producing structures which emerge as a consequence of interacting systems rather than being predetermined. The following books give useful introductions to the field: Mitchell Waldrop (1992), Coveney and Highfield (1995), Johnson (2002) and Buchanan (2001).
3 For further details of Columbo see http://www.columbo-site.freeuk.com/
4 For a full description of the power of the ring see Tolkien (1954: 53–7).
5 See Chapter 5.
6 See Chapter 2.
7 This seems to correspond to Guilbaud et al.'s description of *secondary alexithymia* (Guilbaud, Corcos and Jeammet 2004).

Chapter 9

1 The policy was one which in itself was paradoxical in that in seeking to promote her development through 'normalisation' there was an implicit denial of her individuality – a position which not only goes against psychological processes of individuation but also against ideas central to human rights discourse. I have argued elsewhere (Sutton 2005) that there is a mistake akin to the 'epidemiological fallacy' in pursuing a population-orientated aim to individuals: misapplied to the individual, social inclusion policies can be a form of child abuse through subjecting children to environments for which they are not equipped.

Chapter 10

1 The Milan approach is a structured iterative consultation process. Available information is used to generate hypotheses which are tested in consultations. The hypotheses are developed through discussion between the therapists separately from the family: the approach has similarities to the eight-step PBL model described in Chapter 2. The further information generated is then used to reformulate hypotheses. At the end a formulation is then presented to the family. Each individual is addressed, reflecting back aspects of family life using examples from the clinic contact and history. See Palazzoli et al. (1978), Campbell, Draper and Huffington (1992) and Boston (2000).
2 My clinical experience of family violence, including murder, lead me to think it can be very easy to miss the fact that the 'dynamics of desperation' are operative rather than (or

alongside) sadistic impulses. See Gilligan (2000) for a detailed description and an appreciation of the place of shame in precipitating violence.

3   For debate on these issues see Morrison (1997), Meissner (2002) and Peterson (2002).

Chapter 11

1   We viewed this as the shift from an essential and exceptional 'primary surgical preoccupation' to an essential but ordinary 'primary maternal preoccupation' after Winnicott (1956a).

2   For an extremely clinically useful children's book which captures this see *There's no such thing as a dragon* (Kent 2010).

3   ICD–10 'Individuals who are convinced that they have an abnormality or disfigurement of a specific bodily (often facial) part, which is not objectively noticed by others (sometimes termed dysmorphophobia), should be classified under hypochondriacal disorder (F45.2) or delusional disorder (F22.0), depending upon the strength and persistence of their conviction' (World Health Organisation 2007: 114).

4   Public Accounts Committee 26th report. *Management of NHS hospital productivity*. March 2011. Available at: http://www.publications.parliament.uk/pa/cm201011/cmselect/cmpubacc/741/74102.htm

5   See the 'Head to Head' feature article in Bevan (2009) and Gubb (2009).

6   See Dyer (2011).

7   For descriptions and definitions see: National Leadership and Innovation Agency for Healthcare (2005), NHS Scotland (2007) and Royal College of Nursing (2012).

8   A simple Google search – "Toyota Management System"+description – will give readers 31,500 sites to explore! (3 March 2012).

BIBLIOGRAPHY

Abram J. (1996) *The language of Winnicott: a dictionary of Winnicott's use of words.* London: Karnac Books.

Anon (1908) *The Westminster Review* 18.

Baier A. (1986) Trust and antitrust. *Ethics* 96.2: 231–60.

Balint M. (1957) *The doctor, his patient and the illness.* London: Pitman Medical.

Beck, A. T., Schuyler D. and Herman I. (1974). Development of suicidal intent scales. In A.T. Beck, H. L. P . Resnik and D. Lettieri, eds, *The prediction of suicide.* Charles Press.

Bettelheim B. (1985) *Freud and Man's Soul.* London: Fontana Paperbacks.

Bevan G. (2009) Have targets done more harm than good in the English NHS? No ... *BMJ* 338. doi: 10.1136/bmj.a3129

Bion W. (1957). Differentiation of the psychotic from the non-psychotic personalities. *Int.J.PsychoAnal* 38: 266–75; and in *Second Thoughts.* New York: Aronson (revised 1967).

Blomberg B. (1996) Foreword to Coveney P. and Highfield R. *Frontiers of complexity: the search for order in a chaotic world.* New York: Fawcett Columbine.

Borrell-Carrió F., Suchman A. L. and Epstein R. M. (2004) The biopsychosocial model 25 years later: principles, practice, and scientific inquiry. *Annals of Family Medicine* 2: 576–82.

Boston Children's Hospital/Harvard Medical School http://www.childrenshospital.org/az/ Site2187/mainpageS2187P0.html (accessed 26 October 2011).

Boston P. (2000) Systemic family therapy and the influence of post-modernism. *Advances in Psychiatric Treatment* 6: 450–7. doi: 10.1192/apt.6.6.450

Bowlby J. (1977) The making and breaking of affectional bonds. I. Aetiology and psychopathology in the light of attachment theory. An expanded version of the Fiftieth Maudsley Lecture, delivered before the Royal College of Psychiatrists, 19 November 1976. *British Journal of Psychiatry* 130: 201–210. doi: 10.1192/bjp.130.3.201

Brandell J. R. (1992) Countertransference phenomena in the psychotherapy of children and adolescents. Chapter 1 in *Countertransference in psychotherapy of children and adolescents.* Brandell J. R., ed. Northvale, NJ and London: Jason Aronson Inc.

Buchanan M. (2001) *Ubiquity: the new science that is changing the world.* London: Phoenix.

Campbell D., Draper R. and Huffington C. (1992) *Second thoughts on the theory and practice of the Milan approach to family therapy.* London: Karnac Books.

Christie D. (2000) Cognitive-behavioural therapeutic techniques for children with eating disorders. Chapter 11 in Lask B. and Bryant-Waugh R. (2000) *Anorexia nervosa and related eating disorders in childhood and adolescence.* 2nd edn. Hove: Psychology Press.

Concise Oxford Dictionary (1982) Oxford: Clarendon Press.

Coveney, P. and Highfield, R. (1995) *Frontiers of complexity: the search for order in a chaotic world.* New York and London: Faber and Faber.

David T., Patel L., Burdett K. and Rangachari P. (1999) *Problem-based learning in medicine: a practical guide for students and teachers.* London: Royal Society of Medicine Press.

Daws D. (1989) *Through the night: helping parents and sleepless infants.* London: Free Association Books.

—(1999) Child psychotherapy in the baby clinic of a general practice. *Clinical Child Psychology and Psychiatry* 4.1: 9–22.

Day D. (1994) *Tolkien's ring.* London: Harper Collins.

Department of Health (2008) *Code of Practice Mental Health Act 1983.* London: TSO.

Dyer C. (2011) Mid Staffordshire inquiry will advise on dangers of reform and how to avoid them. *BMJ* 343. doi: 10.1136/bmj.d7920

Edgcumbe R. (2000) *Anna Freud: a view of development, disturbance and therapeutic techniques.* London and Philadelphia: Routledge.

Elmhirst S. I. (1996) Foreword to Kahr B. (1996) *D.W. Winnicott: a biographical portrait.* London: Karnac Books.

Engel G. L. (1977) The need for a new medical model: a challenge for biomedicine. *Science* 196.4(286): 129–36.

Engström I. (2002) Consultation–liaison work in paediatric care. *International Congress Series* 1241: 217–20. http://dx.doi.org/10.1016/S0531–5131(02)00809–9 (accessed 7 March 2012).

Fewtrell M., Wilson D. C., Booth I. and Lucas A. (2011) When to wean? How good is the evidence for six months' exclusive breastfeeding. *BMJ* 342: 209–12.

Freud A. (1936) *The Ego and the mechanisms of defence.* London: Karnac Books (revised 1993).

—(1965) *Normality and pathology in childhood: assessments of development.* London: Hogarth Press and the Institute of Psychoanalysis (revised 1989).

—(1970) The symptomatology of childhood: a preliminary attempt at classification. In Ekins R. and Freeman R., eds *Selected Writings* by Anna Freud. Harmondsworth: Penguin, 1998.

—(1974) A psychoanalytic view of developmental psychopathology. In *Writings*, 8: 57–74. New York: International Universities Press. Cited in Yorke C., Wiseberg S. and Freeman T. (1989) *Development and psychopathology: studies in psychoanalytic psychiatry.* New Haven and London: Yale University Press.

—(1980) *Normality and pathology in childhood: assessments of development.* London: Hogarth Press and the Institute of Psychoanalysis.

—(1989) Mental health and illness in terms of internal harmony and disharmony. In Yorke C., Wiseberg S. and Freeman T., eds (1989) *Development and psychopathology: studies in psychoanalytic psychiatry.* New Haven, CT, and London: Yale University Press, Freud S. (1905) *On sexuality: three essays on the theory of sexuality and other works.* Lectures 20 & 21. Pelican Freud Library vol. 7. Harmondsworth: Penguin Books.

—(1916) Lecture 20 in *Introductory lectures on psychoanalysis*, ed., A. Richards (1981). Harmondsworth: Penguin Books.

—(1927) *Introductory lectures on psychoanalysis.* Penguin Freud Library vol. 1 (1981 edn). Harmondsworth: Penguin Books.

—(1933[1932]) The dissection of the psychical personality. *New Introductory Lectures on Psychoanalysis.* Penguin Freud Library vol. 2 (1979 edn). Harmondsworth: Penguin Books.

Fulford K. W. M., Stanghellini G. and Broome M. (2004) What can philosophy do for psychiatry? *World Psychiatry* 3.3: 130–5.

General Medical Council (2006a) Good medical practice: duties of a doctor. *Good Medical Practice*. London: GMC. http://www.gmc-uk.org/guidance/good_medical_practice/duties_of_a_doctor.asp (accessed 19 June 2012).

—(2006b) Good medical practice: teaching and training, appraising and assessing. *Good Medical Practice*. London: GMC. http://www.gmc-uk.org/guidance/good_medical_practice/teaching_training.asp (accessed 19 June 2012).

Gilligan J. (2000) *Violence: reflections on our deadliest epidemic*. London: Jessica Kingsley Publishers.

Gillon R. (1985) *Philosophical medical ethics*. Chichester and New York: John Wiley.

Gleick J. (1987) *Chaos: making a new science*. London: Cardinal.

Goffman E. (1961) *Asylums: essays on the social situation of mental patients and other inmates*. New York: Anchor Books.

Goodman R. (1997) *Child and adolescent mental health services: reasoned advice to commissioners and providers*. Maudsley Discussion Paper No. 4. London: Institute of Psychiatry.

Greenhalgh T. (1999) Narrative based medicine in an evidence based world. *BMJ* 318(7179): 323–5.

Greenhalgh T. and Hurwitz B. (1998) *Narrative based medicine*. BMJ Books.

Groddeck, G. (1920) On the It. In *The meaning of illness*. London: Maresfield Library (revised 1977).

—(1925) The meaning of illness. Chapter 6 in *The meaning of illness: selected psychoanalytic writings by Georg Groddeck*. London: Maresfield Library Karnac Books.

Gubb J. (2009) Have targets done more harm than good in the English NHS? Yes. *BMJ* 338. doi: 10.1136/bmj.a3130

Guilbaud O. (2004) Guilbaud et al's description of secondary alexithymia. Corcos M. and Jeammet P. (2004) Response to 'Features of alexithymia or features of Asperger's syndrome?' by Fitzgerald. *European Child & Adolescent Psychiatry* 13.6: 394. doi: 10.1007/s00787–004–0421–z

Hampton J. R., Harrison M. J., Mitchell J. R., Prichard J. S. and Seymour C. (1975) Relative contributions of history-taking, physical examination, and laboratory investigation to diagnosis and management of medical outpatients. *British Med Journal* 31.2(5969): 486–9. http://www.ncbi.nlm.nih.gov/pubmed/1148666 (accessed 10 February 2012).

Harrison S. (2009) Co-optation, commodification and the medical model: governing UK medicine since 1991. *Public Administration* 87.2: 184–97. doi: 10.1111/j.1467–9299.2008.01752.x

Hinshelwood R. D. (1989) *A dictionary of Kleinian thought*. London: Free Association Books.

HMG (2005) *Mental Capacity Act 2005*. http://www.legislation.gov.uk/ukpga/2005/9/notes/contents (accessed 19 June 2012).

Holder A. (1995) Anna Freud's contribution to the psychoanalytic theory of development. *Journal of Child Psychotherapy* 21.3: 324–46.

Holmes J. (2011a) Transitional object. *B.J.Psychiatry* 198: 423. doi: 10.1192.110.087676

—(2011b) Projective identification. *B.J.Psychiatry* 198: 364. doi: 10.1192/bjp.bp.110.087684

Johnson S. (2002) *Emergence: the connected lives of ants, brains, cities and software*. London: Penguin Books.

Jones E. (1953) *The life and work of Sigmund Freud* (eds Trilling and Marcus 1974). New York: Basic Books.

Keats J. (1821) in *Oxford dictionary of quotations* (2004). 6th edn. Oxford: Oxford University Press.

Kendall T., Taylor C., Bhatti H., Chan M. and Kapur N. (2011) On behalf of the development group. Longer term management of self harm: summary of NICE guidance. *BMJ* 343: 1167–9. doi: 10.1136/bmj.d7073

Kent J. (2010) *There's no such thing as a dragon.* New York: Golden Book Publishing Co.

Kingsbury S. (1996) PATHOS: a screening instrument for adolescent overdose: a research note. *J. Child Psychol. Psychiat.* 37.5: 609–11.

Klerman G. L. (1977) Mental illness, the medical model, and psychiatry. *Journal of Medicine and Philosophy* 2.3: 220–43.

Knowles E., ed., (2004) *Oxford dictionary of quotations* 6th edition. Oxford: Oxford University Press.

Kraemer S. (1983) 'Who will have my tummy ache if I give it up?' *Family Systems Medicine* 1.4: 51–9. doi: 10.1037/h0089641

Kraemer S. and Loader P. (1995) 'Passing through life': alexythymia and attachment disorders. *Journal of Psychosomatic Research* 39: 937–41.

Kris E. (1952) *Psychoanalytic explorations in art.* New York: International Universities Press. Described in Akhtar S. (2009) *Comprehensive dictionary of psychoanalysis.* London: Karnac Books.

Lain-Entralgo P. (1982) *El diagnóstico médico.* Barcelona: Salvat. Cited in Mezzich J. (2002).

Laplanche J. and Pontalis J. B. (1988) *The language of psychoanalysis.* London: Karnac Books and the Institute of Psychoanalysis.

Lask B. and Fosson A. (1989) *Childhood illness: the psychosomatic approach – children talking with their bodies.* Chichester: John Wiley.

Laufer, M. and Laufer, M. E. (1984) *Adolescence and developmental breakdown: a psychoanalytic view.* New Haven: Yale University Press.

— eds., (1989) *Developmental breakdown and psychoanalytic treatment in adolescence: clinical studies.* New Haven and London: Yale University Press.

Lazenbatt A. and Taylor J. (2011) Fabricated or induced illness in children: a rare form of child abuse? www.nspcc.org.uk/Inform/research/briefings/fii_wda83361.html (accessed 8 February 2012).

Lewin R. (1992) *Complexity: life at the edge of chaos.* New York, Oxford, Singapore and Sydney: Maxwell Macmillan International.

Likierman M. (1995) The debate between Anna Freud and Melanie Klein: An historical survey. *Journal of Child Psychotherapy* 21.3: 313–25.

Lipowski Z. J. (1984) What does the word 'psychosomatic' really mean? A historical and semantic inquiry. *Psychosomatic Medicine* 46.2: 153–71.

Litt I. F., Cuskey, W. R. and Rudd, S. (1983). Emergency room evaluation of the adolescent who attempts suicide: Compliance with follow-up. *Journal of Adolescent Health Care* 4.

Magagna J. (2000) Individual Psychotherapy. Chapter 12 in Lask B. and Bryant-Waugh R. (2000) *Anorexia Nervosa and related eating disorders in childhood and adolescence.* 2nd edn. Hove: Psychology Press.

Malan D. H. (1979) *Individual psychotherapy and the science of psychodynamics.* London: Butterworth.

Malle B. F. and Nelson S. E. (2003) Judging mens rea: the tension between folk concepts and legal concepts of intentionality. *Behavioral Sciences and the Law* 21: 563–80. Published online at Wiley InterScience, www.interscience.wiley.com (accessed 27 December 2011). doi: 10.1002/bsl.554

Mann K., Gordon J. and MacLeod A. (2007) Reflection and reflective practice in health professions education: a systematic review. *Advances in Health Sciences Education* 14.4: 595–621.

Martyn C. (2011) Lactation wars. *BMJ* 342: 362.

McDougall J. (1989) *Theatres of the body: a psychoanalytic approach to psychosomatic illness*. London: Free Association Books.

McFadyen A. (1994) *Special care babies and their developing relationships*. London and New York: Routledge.

McGinn C. (1999) *The mysterious flame: conscious minds in a material world*. New York: Basic Books.

Meissner W. W. (2002) The problem of self-disclosure in psychoanalysis. *J Am Psychoanal Assoc* 50.3: 827–67. doi: 10.1177/00030651020500031501 http://apa.sagepub.com/content/50/3/827

Meltzer D. (1967) *The psycho-analytical process*. Perthshire: Clunie Press.

Menzies Lyth I. (1960) Social systems as a defence against anxiety. *Human Relations* 13: 95–121.

—(1988) *Containing anxiety in institutions: selected essays, Volume 1*. London: Free Association Books.

Merriam, S. B., Caffarella R. S. and Baumgartner L. M. (2007) *Learning in adulthood: A comprehensive guide (3rd ed.)*. Hoboken, NJ: John Wiley.

Mezzich, J. (2002) The WPA international guidelines for diagnostic assessment. *World Psychiatry* 1(1): 36. http://www.ncbi.nlm.nih.gov/pmc/articles/PMC1525053/ (accessed 20 February 2012).

Miller L., Rustin M., Rustin M. and Shuttleworth J. (1989) *Closely observed infants*. London: Duckworth.

Mitchell Waldrop M. (1992) *Complexity: the emerging science at the edge of order and chaos*. London: Penguin Books.

Morrison A. L. (1997) Ten years of doing psychotherapy while living with a life-threatening illness: self-disclosure and other ramifications. *Psychoanalytic Dialogues* 7.2: 225–41. http://www.tandfonline.com/action/showCitFormats?doi=10.1080%2F10481889709539178

Murray A. (2011) Herchel Smith Professor of Molecular Genetics, Harvard University, speaking on BBC Radio 4 *The Life Scientific*, 13 December 2011, via "Transcript" link at: http://www.bbc.co.uk/programmes/b0184rfy#synopsis (accessed 8 March 2012).

Murray L. and Andrews L. (2000) *The social baby: understanding babies' communication from birth*. Richmond, Surrey:. CP Publishing.

Murray L., Arteche A., Fearon P., Halligan S., Goodyer I. and Cooper P. (2011) Maternal postnatal depression and the development of depression in offspring up to 16 years of age. *Journal of the American Academy of Child & Adolescent Psychiatry* 50.5: 460–70. doi: 10.1016/j.jaac.2011.02.001

National Collaborating Centre for Women's and Children's Health (2010) *Constipation in children and young people diagnosis and management of idiopathic childhood constipation in primary and secondary care*. Commissioned by the National Institute for Health and Clinical Excellence, London. http://guidance.nice.org.uk/CG99/Guidance/pdf/English (accessed 19 January 2012).

National Institute for Health & Clinical Excellence (2009a) *Attention deficit hyperactivity disorder: diagnosis and management of ADHD in children, young people and adults*. National Clinical Practice Guideline Number 72. Leicester and London: The British Psychological Society and The Royal College of Psychiatrists. http://guidance.nice.org.uk/CG72/Guidance/pdf/English (accessed 19 June 2012).

—(2009b) *Guideline Development Manual {Online}*. http://www.nice.org.uk/aboutnice/howwework/developingniceclinicalguidelines/clinicalguidelinedevelopmentmethods/GuidelinesManual2009.jsp?domedia=1&mid=60B7B3CD-BBC2-E1BE-A6D53FD68D8845AD (accessed 7 March 2012).

National Mental Health Development Unit (2011) *Guidance for health professionals on medically unexplained symptoms (MUS): making sense of symptoms; managing professional uncertainty; building on patient's strengths*. http://www.nmhdu.org.uk/resources/resources/?keywords=&filter=last_updated&order=desc&p=5 (accessed 8 June 2012).

Nemiah J. C. and Sifneos P. E. (1970) Psychosomatic illness: a problem of communication. *Psychotherapy and Psychosomatics* 18: 154–60. doi: 10.1159/000286074

Obholzer A. and Roberts V.Z. (1994) *The unconscious at work: individual and organisational stress in the human services*. London and New York: Routledge

O'Neill O. (2002a) *A question of trust*. Cambridge: Cambridge University Press. Available at http://www.bbc.co.uk/radio4/reith2002 (accessed 12 December 2011).

—(2002b) *Autonomy and trust in bioethics*. Cambridge: Cambridge University Press.

O'Shaughnessy E. (1964) The absent object. In *Key papers from the Journal of Chid Psychotherapy*. P. S. Barrows, ed. Hove and New York: Brunner-Routledge. Originally published *Journal of Chid Psychotherapy* 1.2: 34–43.

Palazzoli S., Boscolo L., Cecchin G. and Prata, G. (1978) *Paradox and counterparadox*. New York: Aronson.

Peterson M. C., Holbrook J. H., Von Hales D., Smith N. L. and Staker L. V. (1992) Contributions of the history, physical examination, and laboratory investigation in making medical diagnoses. *West J. Med.* 156.2: 163–5. http://www.ncbi.nlm.nih.gov/pubmed/1536065 (accessed 10 February 2012).

Peterson, Z. D. (2002) More than a mirror: The ethics of therapist self-disclosure. *Psychotherapy: Theory, Research, Practice, Training* 39.1: 21–31. psycnet.apa.org/journals/pst/39/1/21.html (accessed 5 March 2012). doi: 10.1037/0033–3204.39.1.21

Philips A. and Taylor B. (2009) *On kindness*. London: Hamish Hamilton.

Psychoanalytic Psychotherapy (2009) Special issue: depressive disorders in the life-cycle: biology, environment and internal world.

PubMed Health (2010) Hydatidiform mole. http://www.ncbi.nlm.nih.gov/pubmedhealth/PMH0001907/ (accessed 8 June 2012).

Raphael-Leff J. (1991) *Psychological processes of childbearing*. London: Chapman and Hall.

Renfrew M. J., McGuire W. and McCormick F. M. (2011) Analysis article was misleading. *BMJ* 342: 399–400.

Robertson J. and Robertson J. (1989) *Separation and the very young*. London: Free Association Books.

Roshan M. and Rao A. P. (2000) A study on relative contributions of the history, physical examination and investigations in making medical diagnosis. *J Assoc Physicians India* 48.8: 771–75. http://www.ncbi.nlm.nih.gov/pubmed/11273467 (accessed 10 February 2012).

Royal College of Nursing (2003) *Restraining, holding still and containing children and young people: guidance for nursing staff*. London: Royal College of Nursing.

Royal College of Psychiatrists (1998) *Managing deliberate self-harm in young people: Council Report CR64*. London: Royal College of Psychiatrists. www.rcpsych.ac.uk/files/pdfversion/cr64.pdf (accessed 1 March 2012).

—(2008) *A competency based curriculum for specialist training in psychiatry: specialist module in child and adolescent psychiatry*. London: Royal College of Psychiatrists. http://www.rcpsych.ac.uk/training/curriculum2010.aspx (accessed 7 March 2012).

—(2009) *Child and adolescent mental health problems in the emergency department and the services to deal with them: Royal College of Psychiatrists Council Report*. Child and Adolescent Faculty of The Royal College of Psychiatrists, Royal College of Paediatrics and Child Health, and British Association of Emergency Medicine and College of Emergency Medicine.

http://www.bing.com/search?q=%22Child+and+Adolescent+Mental+Health+Problems+ in+The+Emergency+Department+and+the+Services+to+Deal+with+them%22&r=834 (accessed 1 March 2012).

—(2011) *Faculty of Liaison Psychiatry* http://www.rcpsych.ac.uk/specialties/faculties/liaison. aspx (accessed 20 June 2012).

Sackett D. L., Rosenberg W. C., Muir Gray J. A., Haynes R. B. and Richardson W. S. (1996) Evidence based medicine: what it is and what it isn't. *BMJ* 312: 71–2.

Segal H. (1981) *The Work of Hanna Segal: A Kleinian approach to clinical practice.* Aronson. Reprinted Free Association Books/Maresfield Library, 1986.

—(1988) *Introduction to the work of Melanie Klein.* London: Karnac Books and the Institute of Psychoanalysis.

Sharpe E. F. (1940) Psycho-physical problems revealed in language: an examination of metaphor. Chapter VII in *Collected papers on psycho-analysis.* Marjorie Brierley, ed. London: Hogarth Press and the Institute of Psychoanalysis.

Shoenberg P. (2007) *Psychosomatics: the uses of psychotherapy.* Basingstoke and New York: Palgrave Macmillan.

Sinason V. (1992) *Mental handicap and the human condition: new approaches from the Tavistock.* London: Free Association Books.

Stern D. (1985) *The interpersonal world of the infant: a view from psychoanalysis and developmental psychology.* London and New York: Karnac Books.

—(1990) Presentation at the conference 'The Effect of relationships on relationships' sponsored by the World Association of Infant Psychiatry, the Tavistock Clinic, and the Anna Freud Centre, London, November.

Stirrat G. M. and Gill R. (2005) Autonomy in medical ethics after O'Neill. *J. Med Ethics* 31: 127–30.

Sutton A. (1987) Dangerous building keep out: an account of a psychotic girl's psychotherapy. *J. Child Psychotherapy* 13.1: 57–76.

—(1997) Authority, autonomy, responsibility and authorisation: with specific reference to adolescent mental health practice. *Journal of Medical Ethics* 23.1: 26–31.

—(1998a) "Lesley": the struggle of a teenager with an intersex disorder to find an identity – its impact on the "I" of the beholder. Chapter 13 (D) in *A stranger in my own body: atypical gender identity development and mental health.* di Ceglie D. and Freedman D., eds. London: Karnac Books.

—(1998b) Psychodynamics of self directed destructive behaviour in adolescence. *Advances in Psychiatric Treatment* 4: 31–8.

—(2001a) Disrupted dependence and dependability: Winnicott in a culture of symptom intolerance. *Psychoanalytic Psychotherapy* 15.1: 1–19.

—(2001b) Consent, latency and psychotherapy or 'What am I letting myself in for?' *Journal of Child Psychotherapy* 27.3: 319–33.

—(2002) Psychoanalytic psychotherapy in paediatric liaison: a diagnostic and therapeutic tool. *Journal of Child Psychotherapy* 28.2: 181–200.

—(2005) Can social inclusion practices be abusive? The non-facilitating educational environment, aggression and 'Forest Fire' children. *First European conference on Child and Adolescent Mental Health in Educational Settings*, 22–23 September 2005, Maison de la Chimie, Paris, France. A Tavistock Clinic Conference in partnership with Association de Psychiatrie de l'Enfant et de l'Adolescent et des Professions Associées, France & University of Naples, Italy.

—(2008) When violence in adults' behaviour puts children at risk: a child psychiatric perspective. Chapter 5 in *Domestic violence: a multi-professional approach for health professionals.* Keeling J. and Mason T., eds. London: Open University Press.

—(2010) Nature and nurture: the gene genie. *Child Concern newsletter*, Manchester. Child Concern.

—(2011) General practitioners' conflicts of interest, the paramountcy principle and safeguarding children: a psychodynamic contribution. *Journal of Medical Ethics* 37: 254–7. doi: 10.1136/jme.2010.040394

—and Hughes L. (2005) The psychotherapy of parenthood: towards a formulation and valuation of concurrent work with parents. *J. Child Psychotherapy* 31.2: 169–88 .

—and Whitaker J. (1998) Intersex disorder in childhood and adolescence: gender identity, gender role, sex assignment and general mental health. Chapter 11 in *A stranger in my own body: atypical gender identity development and mental health.* di Ceglie D. and Freedman D, eds. London: Karnac Books.

Symington N. (1986) *The analytic experience: lectures from the Tavistock.* London: Free Association Books.

Tan N., Sutton A. and Dornan T. (2010) Morality and the philosophy of medicine and education. In Dornan et al., *A Textbook of Medical Education.* Edinburgh: Elsevier.

Taylor E. A. and Stansfeld S. A. (1984). Children who poison themselves. I. A clinical comparison with psychiatric controls. *British Journal of Psychiatry* 145: 127–35 cited in Kingsbury S. (1996).

Tennyson, Alfred Lord. *In Memoriam A.H.H. XXVII.*

Tolkien J. R. R. (1954) *The Fellowship of the Ring.* Book 1 of *The Lord of the Rings* (edition 1994). London: Harper Collins.

Trevarthen C. and Aitken K. J. (1994) Brain development, infant communication, and empathy disorders: intrinsic factors in child mental health. *Development and Psychopathology* 6.4: 579–633.

Ultimate Columbo Site (2012) http://www.columbo-site.freeuk.com/ (accessed 3 March 2012).

Vygotsky L. S. (1978) *Mind and society: the development of higher psychological processes.* Cambridge, MA: Harvard University Press.

Wall P. (1999). *Pain: the science of suffering.* London: Weidenfeld & Nicolson.

Walsh P. C., Retik A. B., Stamey T. A., Darracott Vaughan E., Jr., eds, (1992) *Campbell's Urology, Sixth Edition.* Philadelphia: WB Saunders Co. Cited John Hopkins University Dept of Paediatric Urology. http://urology.jhu.edu/pediatric/diseases/DEx2.php (accessed 26 October 2011).

Webster's Dictionary (1993) Merriam Webster's Collegiate. Springfield, MA: Merriam.

Williams A. F. and Prentice A. (2011) Response: Scientific Advisory Committee on Nutrition replies to Mary Fewtrell and colleagues. *BMJ* 342: 400.

Winnicott D. W. (1951) Transitional objects and transitional phenomena. In *Through paediatrics to psycho-analysis.* London: Hogarth Press and the Institute of Psychoanalysis, pp. 229–42 (revised 1982).

—(1953). Symptom tolerance in paediatrics. In *Through Paediatrics to PsychoAnalysis.* London: Hogarth Press and the Institute of Psychoanalysis (revised 1982).

—(1956a) Primary maternal preoccupation. Chapter XXIV in *Through Paediatrics to Psycho-Analysis.* London: Hogarth Press and the Institute of Psychoanalysis (revised 1982).

—(1956b). The antisocial tendency. In *Through paediatrics to psycho-analysis.* London: Hogarth Press and the Institute of Psychoanalysis (revised 1975).

—(1958) The capacity to be alone. Chapter 2 in *The maturational processes and the facilitating environment: studies in the theory of emotional development*. London: Hogarth Press and the Institute of Psychoanalysis (revised 1965).

—(1962) The aims of psychoanalytic treatment. Chapter 15 in *The maturational processes and the facilitating environment: studies in the theory of emotional development*. London: Hogarth Press and the Institute of Psychoanalysis (revised 1965).

—(1963a) Dependence in infant-care, in child-care and in the psycho-analytic setting. *The maturational processes and the facilitating environment: studies in the theory of emotional development*. London: Hogarth Press and the Institute of Psychoanalysis (revised 1965).

—(1963b) The development of the capacity for concern. Chapter 6 in *The maturational processes and the facilitating environment: studies in the theory of emotional development*. London: Hogarth Press and the Institute of Psychoanalysis (revised 1965).

—(1964) *The child, the family, and the outside world*. Harmondsworth: Penguin Books.

—(1971a) *Therapeutic consultations in child psychiatry*. London: Hogarth Press and the Institute of Psychoanalysis.

—(1971b). *Playing and reality*. New York: Penguin Books.

—(1989) Psycho-somatic illness in its positive and negative aspects. In *Psychoanalytic explorations*. C. Winnicott, R. Shepherd and M. Davis (eds). Cambridge, MA: Harvard University Press.

World Health Organisation (2007) *The ICD–10 classification of mental and behavioural disorders: clinical descriptions and diagnostic guidelines*. http://www.who.int/classifications/icd/en/ (accessed 20 February 2012).

Wright C. (2011) Infection more important than anaemia or allergy. *BMJ* 342: 400.

Xeniditis K., Russell A. and Murphy D. (2001) Management of people with challenging behaviour. *Advances in Psychiatric Treatment* 7: 109–116. doi: 10.1192/apt.7.2.109

Yorke C., Wiseberg S. and Freeman T., eds, (1989) *Development and psychopathology: studies in psychoanalytic psychiatry*. New Haven, CT and London: Yale University Press.

Zinn W. (1993) The empathic physician. *Archives Internal Medicine* 153.3: 306–312.

INDEX